# About the Authors

**Keith Sherwood** is a master of the four classical yogas. He is the author of eight books on energy work, healing and transcendent relationship. The exercises, mudras, and meditations that he has developed are used throughout Europe and North America by healers and energy practitioners to heal physical disease, deep traumas, karmic wounds, and energetic blockages. His ability to see and analyze subtle energy fields has been instrumental in helping people heal relationships and achieve their spiritual goals. Visit Keith on Facebook and at www.onewholelove.com.

**Sabine Wittmann** was born in Salzburg, Austria and graduated from Heilpraktiker (Natural Healer) School in Munich, Germany. In 1997 she opened a private practice for energy healing in Berlin. She has been giving lectures and seminars, as well as writing articles, in Germany and Austria for over ten years.

She currently specializes in women's issues, focusing particularly on the psychological and energetic issues surrounding fertility. As a practitioner of energy work, homeopathy, and several whole body therapies, she has seen first-hand how conditioning and subtle cultural prejudices still adversely affect the energetic and physical health of women. Her goal is to help modern woman to become more creative, radiant, joyful, and free.

## To Write to the Authors

If you wish to contact the author or would like more information about this book, please write to the author in care of Llewellyn Worldwide Ltd. and we will forward your request. Both the author and publisher appreciate hearing from you and learning of your enjoyment of this book and how it has helped you. Llewellyn Worldwide Ltd. cannot guarantee that every letter written to the author can be answered, but all will be forwarded. Please write to:

Keith Sherwood and Sabine Wittmann
⁒ Llewellyn Worldwide
2143 Wooddale Drive
Woodbury, MN 55125-2989
Please enclose a self-addressed stamped envelope for reply,
or $1.00 to cover costs. If outside the U.S.A., enclose
an international postal reply coupon.

Many of Llewellyn's authors have websites with additional information and resources. For more information, please visit our website at http://www.llewellyn.com

# ENERGY HEALING

## for Women

Meditations, Mudras,
*and* Chakra Practices
*to* Restore Your
Feminine Spirit

Keith Sherwood
*AND* Sabine Wittmann

Llewellyn Publications
Woodbury, Minnesota

First Edition
Second Printing, 2015

Cover art: iStockphoto.com/31663566/©stereohype
Cover design: Ellen Lawson
Editing: Gabrielle Rose Simons
Interior illustrations: Mary Ann Zapalac
Interior photographs provided by Keith Sherwood

Llewellyn is a registered trademark of Llewellyn Worldwide Ltd.

**Library of Congress Cataloging-in-Publication Data**
Sherwood, Keith.
  Energy healing for women : meditations, Mudras, and Chakra practices to restore your feminine spirit / Keith Sherwood and Sabine Wittmann. — First Edition.
      pages     cm
  Includes bibliographical references and index.
  ISBN 978-0-7387-4112-3
  1. Energy medicine. 2. Chakra. 3. Meditation. 4. Women—Health and hygiene. 5. Self-care, Health. I. Title.
  RZ999.S5415 2015
  615.8'52082—dc23
                              2015017447

Llewellyn Worldwide Ltd. does not participate in, endorse, or have any authority or responsibility concerning private business transactions between our authors and the public.
    All mail addressed to the author is forwarded but the publisher cannot, unless specifically instructed by the author, give out an address or phone number.
    Any Internet references contained in this work are current at publication time, but the publisher cannot guarantee that a specific location will continue to be maintained. Please refer to the publisher's website for links to authors' websites and other sources.

Llewellyn Publications
A Division of Llewellyn Worldwide Ltd.
2143 Wooddale Drive
Woodbury, MN 55125-2989
www.llewellyn.com

Printed in the United States of America

## Other Books by Keith Sherwood

*The Art of Spiritual Healing*

*Chakra Healing and Karmic Awareness*

*Chakra Therapy*

*Sex and Transcendence*

# Contents

# List of Exercises

# List of Illustrations

# *Prologue*

You have unlimited resources of power, creativity, and radiance within you. In *Energy Healing for Women*, you will learn how to use your unlimited power to heal yourself on the levels of body, soul, and spirit—in the human energy field—at the root of disease.

*Energy Healing for Women* was written for two reasons. First, to show you how to heal karmic patterns and physical ailments that have prevented you from experiencing the entire spectrum of radiant good health, vitality, and intimate relationships. And second, to help those of you who are ready to experience a deeper liberation and joy to expand your boundaries, so that you can experience new worlds within yourself of unlimited peace, power, and freedom.

You can experience these new worlds within you regardless of your present circumstances by using the healing techniques in this book. External changes may appear difficult at the moment. However, at the end of the day, it's the internal changes you make which are the most important and the most enduring. That's because everything you need, including the consciousness, energy, and creative power to heal yourself on the levels of your body, soul, and spirit, is already within you.

In *Energy Healing for Women* you will use the techniques of chakra healing, karmic release, and raja yoga, as well as massage, mudras, dance, meditation, and affirmations to liberate your body, soul, and spirit once and for all.

In each chapter, we will delve into an important energetic issue that has limited your power, creativity, and/or radiance. We will analyze it on both the physical level and subtle levels of energy and consciousness. Then we will provide you with a series of simple exercises designed to heal the issue as quickly as possible.

In one simple technique, you will learn to increase your self-confidence by loving your unloved body parts. In another, you will learn to use your functions of mind to overcome restrictive patterns. You will learn to create life-affirming archetypes that will increase your self-confidence and inner strength. Two chapters have been devoted to chakra healing and healing karmic wounds. Another chapter is devoted to enhancing both inner beauty and physical radiance, something a woman can do at any age. Special attention has been given to healing the wounds you suffered from past life and early childhood traumas, as well as the trauma many women suffered from the loss of an unborn child during pregnancy.

You will learn to create a healing space that you can use to heal yourself and the people you love. You will learn simple techniques to enhance your intuition, creativity, and sensuality. Since spiritual healing is not complete unless you've found your dharma (purpose and life path), we've provided you with a simple regimen that will enable you to cut through the static and find it. Finally, you will learn to make the transition from a traditional relationship to a transcendent relationship and to share what you've learned with your family and circle of friends.

What makes *Energy Healing for Women* different from other books is that you will learn to heal wounds, traumas, and karmic patterns at their root, in your subtle energy system. By taking control of your own healing and getting to the root of your issues you will experience firsthand that everything you need for a joyful, satisfying life is already within you.

Sabine and Keith have been together for fifteen years, and have more than thirty years of experience working with women and men of all ages, in North America, Europe, and Africa.

Keith Sherwood is a master of the four classical yogas. He is the author of seven books on energy work, healing, and transcendent relationships. The exercises, mudras, and meditations that he has developed are used throughout Europe and North America by healers and energy practitioners to heal physical disease, deep traumas, karmic wounds, and energetic blockages. His ability to see and analyze subtle energy fields has been instrumental in helping people achieve their spiritual goals. Visit Keith at www.onewholelove.com and on Facebook at Keith Sherwood—Onewholelove.

Sabine Wittmann is an alternative healer and energy master who uses bodywork, acupuncture, reflexology, and homeopathy to heal women. Her empathy and advanced healing techniques have helped women overcome reproductive issues, early childhood traumas, and relationship issues that bear directly on a woman's self-esteem and personal life path (dharma). Visit Sabine at www.awomanshealingspace.com.

# ONE

## The Universal Feminine

After emerging from Universal Consciousness, creative feminine energy began to function as the driving force of evolution. It's feminine energy emerging from every corner of the universe and from every female of every species that provides the power to create and procreate.

Feminine energy is universal and life-affirming. It motivates humans to unite and to experience intimacy with one another. It can never be taken away from you, and because of that, it makes everybody a healer, a lover, and on the deepest level a radiant, transcendent being who has the capacity to transform the world through their work and relationships.

Although women and men are experiencing a Renaissance of freedom and self-awareness in the twenty-first century, if you look deep enough within yourself you will find a karmic legacy that has prevented you from becoming the person you're capable of being. This legacy exists in the subtle blockages you carry in your energy field, the subtle field of energy and consciousness that exists within you and surrounds you on all dimensions.

We will talk about the subtle energy field at greater length later in this book. For now it's important that you know that your energy field is composed of energetic vehicles that allow you to express yourself and interact with your environment on both the physical and non-physical levels. It also contains resource fields and a subtle energy system that supplies your energy field with life-affirming, feminine energy.

It's the subtle energetic blockages in a person's energy field, and the restrictive patterns they create, that explains why, even with all the freedom people have today, many people have difficulty reaching their full potential, a potential that is fully developed at birth and which the ancient masters of yoga and tantra taught would emerge and blossom through the various stages of life.

## Life-Affirming Energy

*Energy Healing for Women* was designed as a practical book that you can use to heal yourself and the people you love on the levels of soul, spirit, and body. In the chapters that follow, you will learn to perform simple exercises to access the unlimited bounty of life-affirming feminine energy within you. You will also learn to share your feminine energy freely with those you love and those who will benefit from your healing. Life-affirming, feminine energy is the foundation of a woman's power, creativity, and radiance. This energy can be enhanced in every woman. The energy we're talking about goes by many names and has been venerated in many societies. Taoists in China call it Chi or Ki. In India, it's called Prana and Shakti. It doesn't matter what name it goes by; this extraordinary energy can be used to heal trauma and physical disease. It can be used to heal restrictive patterns that limit you and disrupt your relationships. And, most importantly, because it only has universal qualities, it can be used to heal your soul and spirit on the deepest levels so that you can experience the transcendent love and joy that is your birthright.

## Universal Qualities of the Feminine

The universal qualities of the feminine include healing and the power, creativity, and radiance that support it. They also include pleasure, love, intimacy, joy, and the qualities of good character, which for millennia have been embraced by women of all cultures. These qualities include non-harming, loyalty, perseverance, discipline, patience, long-suffering, and courage. Knowing yourself as an expression of the universal feminine will empower you to be your "Self" and share your self in your fullness.

In fact, by integrating this life-affirming energy into your everyday life and celebrating its universal qualities, alone or with your partner, you will affirm the truth that "Women are Gods, women are life, women are adornment." These words of Dr. John Mumford, in *Ecstasy Through Tantra* were attributed to the Buddha.

## The Ancestral Women

You may not be aware of it, but enhancing and celebrating the universal qualities of the feminine has been central to the customs of many traditional societies. Although the vast majority disappeared long ago or were absorbed into more dominant societies, those that remain cling to a remnant of their ancestral customs.

In today's world, the largest group of people who maintain these ancient traditions are the Minangkabau of Sumatra. At three million, the Minangkabau are one of the few societies that have taken pains to preserve the customs that balance the needs of women and men and that seek openly to enhance the life-affirming qualities of the universal feminine.

Societies such as the Minangkabau are matriarchal. They provide a resource for women who seek to heal their body, soul, and spirit and to share their natural feminine power, creativity, and radiance more freely.

Matriarchal societies were once abundant throughout the world, and women living in them were treated as precious jewels because they personified the qualities of the universal feminine.

## The Precious Jewel

This truth is reflected even today in the Indian tradition of the Devadassi. Traditionally, these Indian priestesses had the ability to heal others with their dance because they were taught to freely radiate the pure essence of feminine energy, which grants life, as well as healing. One way that the Devadassi enhanced and celebrated the precious jewel was by using mudras in their dance and in healing.

A mudra is a symbolic gesture that can be made with the hands and fingers or in combination with the tongue and feet. The word *mudra* comes from the Sanskrit root *mud*, which means "delight" or "pleasure."

Although new to the Western world, mudras have been used in the East for centuries to enhance the physical, mental, emotional, and spiritual well-being. Taoists in Ancient China used them to find inner peace; Indian mystics used them to attain samadhi (enlightenment); and healers have used them to heal everything from headaches to arthritis.

Mudras work because they stimulate the flow of subtle energy, prana-chi, through specific energetic centers and meridians in the subtle energy system. By stimulating these points for extended periods of time, usually for five minutes or more, it's possible to release blocked energy that can heal self-limiting and destructive patterns and lead to enhanced levels of self-awareness.

Like the Devadassi, you can liberate the precious jewel within you by performing the Precious Jewel Mudra. We developed the Precious Jewel Mudra because the precious jewel has a direct connection to the Kundalini-Shakti. The Kundalini-Shakti is the greatest repository of feminine energy in the human body. Therefore it represents a source of inner strength and confidence for everyone who is ready to embrace the universal qualities of the feminine. By awakening the precious jewel within you, you will be taking a significant step toward experiencing the ancient power, creativity, and radiance of the universal feminine within you.

## Exercise: The Precious Jewel Mudra

To perform the Precious Jewel Mudra, sit in a comfortable position with your back straight. Then bring your tongue to the top of your mouth and slide it back until the hard palate becomes soft. Hold it there while you put the soles of your feet together. Bring the outside of your index fingers together from the tips to the first joint. Then bring the tips of your middle fingers together to create a triangle. Curl your ring fingers into the palm next. And bring the outside of the ring fingers together so that they're touching from the first to the second joint. Bring the tips of your pinkies together to form another triangle. Then lay your left thumb in the cradle created by your right index finger and lay your right thumb in the cradle created by your left index finger

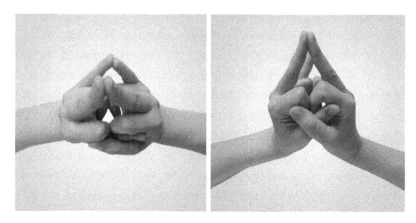

*Figure 1: The Precious Jewel Mudra*

Close your eyes and hold the mudra for ten minutes. In a short time you will feel that your center of awareness emerges from a point deep inside you. This is the precious jewel.

Don't do anything after you've made contact with it. You will receive more benefits from the mudra if you give up all striving and let the Precious Jewel Mudra lead you into a deeper recognition of your innate power and radiance.

You can use the Precious Jewel Mudra as part of your regular regimen of energy work or whenever you seek to increase your self-confidence and inner strength.

## The Growing Child

From the masters of tantra we've learned that children, until they reach the age of seven, naturally celebrate the universal qualities of the feminine, represented by the precious jewel. However, as they grow older, the natural celebration of these qualities can be disrupted.

The disruption we're referring to is not confined to the physical plane. Humans are inter-dimensional beings, and a growing child can become the target of negative influences on the non-physical dimensions.

These negative influences come in the form of energetic projections from other people and karmic baggage—the dense, self-limiting energy that everyone carries with them, in their subtle energy field, from one lifetime to another. We will talk more about these themes later. For now, it's important to recognize that children are particularly susceptible to these influences as they grow older and their ego emerges and begins to dominate their life. They assimilate the cultural values that devalue them and as they become more attached to fields of subtle, non-physical energy that block the natural flow of life-affirming, feminine energy through their body and the energy field that that fills it and extends beyond it.

It's true that it's life-affirming feminine energy which brings pleasure, love, intimacy, and joy into a each person's life, and it's this same energy that provides the medium through which people can share this energy with anyone else ready and open to receive it.

## Cassandra

In Greek mythology, the tragic story of Cassandra illustrates this point clearly. Because of her unique qualities, Cassandra, the mythical daughter of King Priam and Queen Hecuba of Troy, was gifted by the god Apollo with the power of prophecy. Unfortunately, when she spurned Apollo's sexual advances, he cursed her and the very qualities that made her an extraordinary woman and attractive to the god of medicine and healing: her beauty, independence, strength, and intelligence led her to her downfall and subsequent death.

## Witch Hunts

Then there is the sordid history of witch hunts in Europe and North America. In the fourteenth century, during and after the bubonic plague (1347–1349), people in central Europe focused their fear and rage on witches and "plague-spreaders," whom they believed were attempting to destroy their neighbors through magic and poison. Witchcraft cases, particularly against women, increased slowly but steadily from the fourteenth–fifteenth century. Then, around 1550, the persecution skyrocketed. As the historian Steven Katz noted, "The overall evidence makes plain that the growth—the panic—in the witch craze was inseparable from the stigmatization of women" (quoted in Jones).

## Women in Modern Society

Fortunately, modern women are no longer cursed by the gods or condemned as witches. In fact, the last two hundred years have seen a transformation in the way society views women. Laws and customs have changed in most advanced technological societies, which means that women's natural aspirations are no longer routinely suppressed and/or frustrated.

What this means is simple: If you embrace the universal qualities of the feminine you will be able to delight in your ability to surrender to intimacy and transcendent relationships. Your decisions will support your goals and your body will become a glowing tribute to the universal feminine.

A woman, regardless of her age, who has brought the precious jewel into her conscious awareness and immersed herself in the universal qualities of the feminine will light up any room she enters. Such a woman will manifest a new femininity in the world that combines the myths that celebrate the universal feminine and the freedom women have achieved in modern Western society.

We call this new woman, who has healed herself and who is a beacon of light and love, the radiant woman.

## You Can Change Your Life

By performing the Precious Jewel Mudra, you took the first step. The next step will be to overcome the fear that blocks your access to your energy field. You will do that by learning to perform the Fearless Mudra. After that, you will use the Self-Acceptance Mudra to accept yourself as you are now.

Once you've completed these steps, all you must do is use what you will learn in the following chapters to heal your body, soul, and spirit.

Rest assured, by learning to make the inner changes first, you will release all the power, energy, and creativity you need, and you will be able to express it all freely.

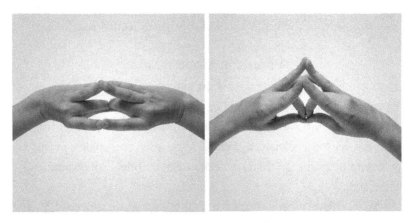

*Figure 2: The Fearless Mudra*

## Exercise: The Fearless Mudra

To perform the Fearless Mudra, find a comfortable position with your back straight. Then bring your tongue to your top palate and slide it back until the hard palate curls upward and softens. Once your tongue is in position, bring the soles of your feet together until they're touching. The index fingers are brought together next so that the tips touch one another. After the tips of your index fingers are touching, bring the tips of your thumbs and the tips of your middle fingers together. Keep the tips of your index fingers above the tips of your thumbs and middle fingers. Then bring the tips of your ring fingers together and the tips of the pinkies together.

Practice the mudra for ten minutes. Then release your fingers and bring your tongue and feet back to their normal positions.

You can use this mudra as part of your regular regimen of energy work or whenever attachments to restrictive beliefs or man-made archetypes use fear to prevent you from freely radiating energy with universal qualities. Repeat as needed.

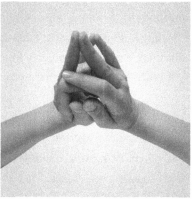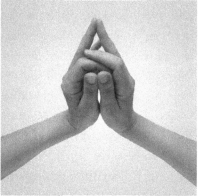

*Figure 3: The Self-Acceptance Mudra*

---

## Exercise: The Self-Acceptance Mudra

The Self-Acceptance Mudra will help you to accept yourself even when you've been trapped by restrictive beliefs or when other people have co-erced you into abandoning your core values to meet their demands.

To perform the mudra, find a comfortable position with your back straight. Then bring your tongue to your top palate and slide it back until the hard palate curls upward and softens. Keep the tip of your tongue in contact with your upper palate while you place the soles of your feet together. Next, bring the mounts of Venus and the edges of your thumbs together. Then slide your right index finger over your left index finger so that the tip of the right finger rests atop the second joint of your left finger. The middle fingers are placed together so that the tips are touching. Once they're touching, place the outsides of the ring fingers together from the first to the second joint. Then bring the inside of the pinkies together from the tips to the first joints.

Practice the mudra for ten minutes. Then release your fingers and bring your tongue and feet back to their normal position. Repeat as needed.

By practicing the Self-Acceptance Mudra regularly, you will be able to accept yourself as you are now and you will bring yourself one step closer to becoming a radiant woman.

## Summary

Like every woman, you have vast amounts of feminine energy lying dormant within you. The process of healing begins when you embrace the universal feminine and liberate this energy, so that it radiates freely through your energy field and physical body. You've done that by performing the Precious Jewel Mudra.

By using the Fearless Mudra to banish fear, you will liberate even more energy. And, by practicing the Self-Acceptance Mudra, you've begun a process that will bring you, step-by-step, closer to achieving your personal and spiritual goals. In the next chapter, you will learn to reclaim your strong center in your physical body and your subtle energy field, and to center yourself in your authentic mind, your authentic vehicle of healing.

## TWO

# Finding Your Strong Center

In the early days of civilization when large villages began to form, women believed that the universal feminine ruled supreme, and that her power and love would maintain the balance between men and women forever. They believed this because they held fast to their strong center, and they trusted the power of the universal feminine. Because of their faith in themselves, their power radiated freely through their subtle energy field and physical body.

Unfortunately, many people don't trust the universal feminine completely; others don't even know that they have vast, untapped reserves of feminine power lying dormant within their subtle energy field. As a result, many people still don't receive all the benefits of the feminine power that radiates through their body, soul, and spirit.

Of course, the idea that someone might not trust the energy that nourishes them may elicit a skeptical response. But consider this: virtually all human beings have lived many lives. And the legacy of their past lives, as well as their distorted relationship to their own feminine power, remains entrenched within their energy field in the form of energetic blockages.

The concept of past lives may seem strange to you if you are new to healing and energy work. But as an inter-dimensional being with a

soul, spirit, and a subtle energy field that supports them, you participate in a grand cycle of life, death, and rebirth.

Although you experience the loss of your physical body at the end
of each life, the energetic vehicles, which are the foundation of your
soul and spirit, live on. At the end of each cycle of life, death, and rebirth, they are incarnated into a new physical body designed to take
them through the next phase of your evolutionary journey. This process continues until you've achieved a permanent state of enlightenment. In the enlightened state you will become fully conscious of your
*a priori* state of bliss and you will transcend the cycle of death and rebirth, which means you will no longer need to be incarnated on earth.

## Man-Women

An extreme example of people who distrust their own feminine power,
and who suffer needlessly, can be found in northern Albania, in one of
the strangest and most enduring institutions in Europe. In this moun-
tainous region, so-called man-women can be found. Man-women are
women who've rejected their feminine power and even their female
identity. These women take on the role of the breadwinner for their
extended family after the patriarch, the father or the elder brother, has
died. According to tradition, the man-woman takes on this role in order
to protect the family from robbery and rape. Unfortunately for these
women, the tradition of man-women demands that they sacrifice a life
as a wife and mother for the sake of their family. Such women abandon
their femininity; they cut their hair short, wear men's clothes, and do
the traditional work of men for the rest of their lives. It's interesting to
note that everyone accepts this obvious deception, including women.
And under normal conditions, a man-woman is treated no differently
than a man by both men and women in the community.

## The Importance of Trust

For those of you who yearn to heal yourselves on the deepest levels, the
man-woman illustrates the importance of trust in both the universal
qualities of the feminine and in yourself. A lack of trust can make it impossible for you to find your strong center. And, without a strong cen-

ter it will be difficult to use your energy field for healing and to unleash all of your potential feminine power. Dreams materialize into physical reality and wishes will come true once you've found your strong center and live within it.

Trust is important for additional reasons. It's self-trust that supports a dynamic, outgoing personality. And, it's trust in yourself and in the universal feminine that will enable you to establish and maintain healthy relationships with yourself and other people.

Fortunately, even if a woman distrusts herself and feminine energy, there are times when it's impossible to block the universal qualities of the feminine completely. Feminine energy and the universal qualities that emerge from it can burst into a woman's conscious awareness and transform her when she is pregnant, when her hormones and enhanced flow of feminine energy make her more radiant. It can overcome a woman's distrust when she has her period and when she meets the love of her life. Especially at the beginning of such an intensive relationship, a woman will find that in order to please her partner, it's impossible to distrust or reject the universal qualities of the feminine completely.

Unfortunately, these bursts of energy are usually temporary. But they need not be. With the help of the exercises that follow you can make feminine energy a permanent part of your life and relationships. The first exercise you will learn to perform is the Trust Mudra. If you perform the Trust Mudra ten minutes a day for at least five days, you will become more receptive to your own feminine energy. That will make it easier for you to trust yourself and to appreciate of the power, creativity and radiance that are your birthright.

---

## Exercise: The Trust Mudra

To perform the Trust Mudra, find a comfortable position with your back straight. Once you're relaxed, bring the tip of your tongue to the top of your mouth. Then slide it back until your upper palate turns soft. Next, bring the soles of your feet together. Continue by bringing your thumbs together so that they're touching each other from the tips to first joint. Bring your index fingers together so that they're touching each other from the tips to first joint. Your thumbs will make a triangle, as will your index fingers. Bring the outside of your remaining three fingers together so that the corresponding fingers in both hands are touching each other from the first to second joint.

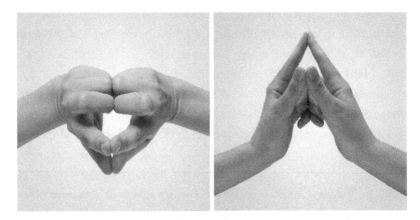

*Figure 4: The Trust Mudra*

Hold the mudra for ten minutes with your eyes closed. After ten minutes, release the mudra and enjoy the enhanced trust you have for yourself and the feminine energy that empowers you. Repeat as needed.

## Finding Your Strong Center

Once you've performed the Trust Mudra, you can reclaim your strong center, first in your physical body, by centering yourself in Hara, and then in your subtle energy field by learning to perform the Standard Method.

Your Hara is located four fingers width below your navel and about one inch (two-and-a-half centimeters) forward from your spine. In Japanese, the word *Hara* means "abdomen." Hara is often linked with another Japanese word, *Tanden*. *Tanden* means "elixir field" (Stiene and Stiene). Hara can therefore be understood to be the place in your physical body where you can find the elixir of life. It is also the place where you can reclaim your powerful center in your physical body.

Most people in the West are unaware of the importance of Hara. That is one reason why so many people still lack all the vitality and healing energy available to them. It also explains why so many people are out of balance, and why they're suspended from a point just above their shoulders and dangle there like puppets. Their physical body, its posture, and the way it moves reflect the fact that they have not made Hara a part of their everyday life.

Problems such as poor posture, chronic muscle tension (which inhibits the flow of prana through the human energy system), compressed and twisted spine, cramped body organs, and poor circulation can be directly linked to being balanced from the shoulders, and not from Hara. Not being centered in your strong center can create additional problems. It can put strain on the joints and ligaments. And that can contribute to mental and physical fatigue and even depression, which is more prevalent in women than men.

So, what is to be gained by Hara? A great deal. Finding your strong center in Hara will empower you. It will connect the energy centers in your abdomen with those in your heart and head. Your reproductive organs will receive more nourishment and will function better. And, by liberating the energy in your abdomen you will have greater access to your deepest emotions and feelings.

Therefore it shouldn't come as a surprise to learn that all major spiritual traditions agree that a solid foundation is a prerequisite for personal growth. Nature itself reflects this principle. For a tree to reach the heavens it must have a solid foundation in the earth. Without this, the tree is liable to remain weak and reactive to each small change in the weather.

---

## Exercise: Hara Breathing

Hara breathing is an ancient technique that has been practiced in the Far East for centuries. It's designed to help people find their strong center in their physical body. If you feel alienated from your body or empty and in need of inner strength, if you feel agitated or overwhelmed, scared or angry, breathing into the Hara will ease these feelings by bringing you back into your strong center and into balance with the rest of the world.

You can practice Hara breathing in any position as long as your back is straight. For now, we suggest you perform Hara breathing while you're lying down on your back. As you progress, you can practice the exercise in a sitting or standing position.

Begin Hara breathing with your arms at your sides, palms up, and your fingers loosely extended. Your eyes should be closed and your jaw kept loose by allowing your mouth to drop open comfortably. From this position, begin breathing deeply through your nose for about three to four minutes. Then bring your mental attention to your Hara, four finger widths below your navel.

Once you've brought your mental attention to Hara, use the middle finger of your positive hand (right hand if you're right-handed, left hand if you're left-handed) to make small clockwise circles around Hara. In a short time, you'll notice sensations emerging from that vital point. You could experience warmth, tingling and/or throbbing sensations, coolness or pressure. None of these sensations should worry you; they're all normal. After a few moments, place both your hands directly on your Hara. At the same time, touch your tongue to your upper palate, directly behind your teeth. This will connect the female and male currents of prana in your energy field and enhance your experience.

Once your hands are in position, you will use the prana entering your energy field on each inhalation to activate your Hara even further. To do that, inhale deeply through the nose into Hara for a count of five. As you fill Hara with prana, visualize that a fluid is flowing in, filling that vital point with energy and light. Retain your breath for a count of five while your mental attention remains focused on Hara. During the retention, as the level of prana increases, you will begin to feel your Hara heating up and your center of balance shifting into vital point.

After you've retained the breath for a count of five, exhale through your mouth for a count of five. There should be no separation between exhalation and the next inhalation. Only in the retention is the natural rhythm broken.

Perform this exercise two to three times a week for about twenty minutes. By mastering hara breathing, you will return to your true center, which is in hara. Repeat as needed.

## Your Strong Center in Your Subtle Energy Field

Now that you've found your strong center in your physical body, you can continue by performing an exercise we call the Standard Method. The Standard Method will enable you to reclaim your strong center in your energy field. After you've performed the Standard Method, you will create a visual screen. The visual screen is an essential part of many of the healing exercises you will learn in this book. Finally, you will learn to perform the Empowerment Mudra. The Empowerment Mudra will help you transmute feminine energy into power once you've found your strong center in your physical body and subtle energy field.

---

## Exercise: The Standard Method

To find your strong center in your energy field, you must be able to focus your mental attention without being distracted. You do that quite naturally whenever you do something you enjoy. Something you enjoy might include reading a book, participating in a lively discussion, or sharing intimacy with someone you love. Enjoyment is the key to success when it comes to focusing the mind and shifting your awareness into your energy field. That's because enjoyment enhances the flow of prana through your energy field and authentic mind.

Your authentic mind is composed of your energy field, your nervous system, and your organs of perception, which can be directed at both your external environment (the physical world) or your internal environment (the subtle worlds of energy and consciousness). It's your authentic mind that is your authentic vehicle of awareness and expression. It's your strong center in the subtle world of energy and consciousness.

The more prana flowing through your energy field and by extension your authentic mind, the easier it will be for you to stay centered and for your awareness to emerge naturally without being distracted.

The Standard Method takes about twenty minutes. In the first part, you will relax the major muscle groups of your physical body by contracting and releasing them. This helps to quiet your mind by releasing residual stress. In the second part, you will use your intent to turn your organs of perception inward so that you can locate and stay centered in your subtle energy field.

It's important to note that in this exercise your *intent* serves the same function as a computer software program. Just as a software program instructs a computer to perform a particular task, your intent instructs your authentic mind to turn your organs of perception inward.

Your organs of perception include your senses, which gather physical-material input, as well as your other, non-physical means of knowing, such as intuition. If you use your intent properly, without watching yourself, trying too hard, or mixing your intent with sentiment and self-doubt, your perception will automatically turn inward.

To begin the Standard Method, find a comfortable position with your back straight. Close your eyes and breathe deeply through your nose for two to three minutes. Then slowly count backward from five to one. As you count backward, mentally repeat and visualize each number three times to yourself. Take your time and let your mind be as creative as it likes. After you reach the number one, repeat this affirmation to yourself: *"I'm now deeply relaxed, feeling better than I did before."*

Continue by counting backward from ten to one, letting yourself sink deeper on each descending number. When you reach the number one, assert, *"Every time I come to this level of mind, I'm able to use more of my mind in more creative ways."*

Next, inhale and bring your attention to your feet. Contract the muscles of your feet as much as possible. Hold your breath for five seconds. Then release your breath and allow the muscles of your feet to relax. Inhale deeply again and repeat the process with your ankles and calves. Continue in the same way with your knees, thighs, buttocks and pelvis, middle and upper abdomen, chest, shoulders, neck, arms and hands. After you've tightened and relaxed all those body parts, squeeze the muscles of your face and hold for five seconds. After five seconds, release and say *"ahh"* as you exhale. Next, open your mouth, stick out your tongue, and stretch the muscles of your face as much as possible. Hold for five seconds. Then release the muscles of your face and say *"ahh"* as you exhale.

Finally, contract your entire body and squeeze the muscles of your face while you hold your breath for five seconds. Expel the breath through your nose and relax for a few moments.

Continue by asserting, *"It's my intent to turn my organs of perception inward."* Take a few moments to enjoy the effects; then assert, *"It's my intent to center myself in my subtle energy field."*

Immediately your orientation will shift, and from your new vantage point, deep within yourself, you will become aware that you are centered in your energy field and authentic mind because you will feel lighter, more yourself and, most importantly, thoughts and feelings will no longer distract you.

Take fifteen minutes more to enjoy the exercise. Then count from one to five and open your eyes. The more often you use the Standard Method, the greater the benefits will be and the easier it will be to stay focused without being distracted. Now that you've found your strong center in your subtle energy field, you can create a visual screen.

---

## Exercise: The Visual Screen

To create a visual screen, find a comfortable position with your back straight. Then close your eyes and relax. To continue, use the Standard Method to relax your physical body and center yourself in your subtle energy field and authentic mind. After you've relaxed your physical body and you're centered, you will create a screen eight feet (two-and-a-half meters) in front of you. The screen should be white and large enough to fit a life sized image of yourself. It should also be raised off the floor so that you must look up at a thirty-degree angle to see the image on the screen clearly.

To create the visual screen, assert, *"It's my intent to visualize a white screen eight feet (two-and-a-half meters) in front of me."* Once the visual screen has materialized, assert, *"It's my intent to visualize an image of myself on the screen."* Immediately, you will see an image of yourself appear on the screen. Observe it for about five minutes. After five minutes, release the image of yourself and release the screen. Then count from one to five and open your eyes.

In the chapters that follow, you will use the visual screen to replace self-limiting archetypes with life-affirming archetypes, to release attachments that block you, and to heal yourself on the levels of body, soul, and spirit. Now that you've created the visual screen, you're ready to perform the Empowerment Mudra.

The Empowerment Mudra is designed to enhance the transmutation of feminine energy into power and to distribute it uniformly throughout your subtle energy field.

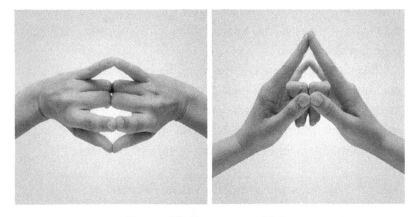

*Figure 5: The Empowerment Mudra*

## Exercise: The Empowerment Mudra

To perform the mudra, find a comfortable position with your back straight. Then use the Standard Method to center yourself in your energy field and authentic mind. By performing the Standard Method first, you will enhance the mudra's effect. Continue by placing the tip of your tongue directly behind the point where your teeth meet your upper gum. Put the outside tips of your thumbs together to form a triangle. Then put the tips of your index fingers together to form the second triangle. Once the tips of your index fingers are touching, put the outside of your middle and ring fingers together from the first to the second joint. Then put the inside tips of your pinkies together to form a third triangle.

When you look down at your hands, you will see three triangles. The first triangle has been created by your thumbs. The second triangle has been created by your index fingers, and the third triangle has been created by your pinkies.

Hold the mudra for ten minutes with your eyes closed. After ten minutes, release the mudra. Then count from one to five and open your eyes. Your will feel wide-awake, perfectly relaxed, and better than before. Repeat as needed.

## Summary

By learning to perform the Trust Mudra and by reclaiming your strong center in your physical body, and in your subtle energy field, you took an important step toward reclaiming your power, creativity, and radiance. By learning to create the visual screen and to perform the Empowerment Mudra, you took an important step in empowering yourself. In the next chapter, you will learn to distinguish the difference between life-affirming feminine energy and the energy that causes suffering and disease. After you've learned that, you will learn to perform chakra healing. By performing chakra healing, you will be able to use the organs of your energy system heal yourself and the people you love.

# THREE

## Chakra Healing

Now that you've reclaimed your strong center in your body and subtle energy field and you've learned to create a visual screen, you can begin the process of chakra healing. By performing chakra healing, you can heal ailments in your body, mind, and soul, as well as in your relationships, at their root, in your subtle energy field.

Before you can begin chakra healing, however, it's important that you recognize two things. First: there are two types of energy in the universe, energy with universal qualities and energy with individual qualities. Second: your subtle energy field and subtle energy system are designed to transmit and transmute energy with universal qualities exclusively. They cannot transmit or transmute energy with individual qualities.

## Energy with Universal Qualities

Energy with universal qualities is responsible for creating the diversity of life that exists in both the physical and non-physical universe. Without it, there would be no awe-inspiring universe, no sentient beings with an energy field and physical body to be aware of it, and no pleasure, love, intimacy, or joy.

Some of you may already recognize the extraordinary power of this energy. You may realize that this force is so powerful that, when it radiates through your energy field freely, it can heal disease and it can catapult you into a state of transcendence where problems and worries disappear and you can participate in the bliss that is continuously experienced by the living universe.

## Energy with Individual Qualities (the Gunas)

We've already talked about energy with universal qualities. This is the original form of feminine energy that emerged when the non-physical universe came into being. However, there is another form of energy that emerged a short time later. This is the energy we perceive through our organs of perception. It has individual qualities and changes continuously.

On the physical level, heat, electricity, and light are good examples of energy with individual qualities. But energy with individual qualities is not confined to the physical level. In the non-physical universe, there are also fields of energy with individual qualities that have what you can think of as character, or what we call a "flavor." You already know this energy. It's the same dense energy that creates pressure and muscle ache when you're stressed and which produces anxiety, self-doubt, and confusion when it's consciously or unconsciously activated. In fact, energy with individual qualities in one form or another is the principal source of both human suffering and physical disease.

The masters of tantra used the gunas to describe the flavor of energy fields with individual qualities. The Sanskrit word *guna* means "quality or attribute." In classical tantra, three gunas known as Sattva, Ragas, and Tamas are used to describe energy with individual qualities.

Tamasic energy is the most dense and distorted form of energy with individual qualities. When there is an inordinate amount of tamasic energy trapped in your subtle energy field, it will cause the most distress and will have the most disruptive effect on your health and well-being.

Ragistic energy is less dense than tamasic energy. In most cases, ragistic energy will have less impact on your health and well-being. But the presence of an inordinate amount of ragistic energy will push you out of your strong center and make it difficult for you to embrace the universal qualities of the feminine.

Sattvic energy is less dense than either tamasic or ragistic energy. This makes it less disruptive to human health and well-being. However, it can still separate you from your strong center in your physical body and subtle energy field. And it can make it difficult for you to be yourself and express yourself freely.

## The Subtle Energy System

Your subtle energy field has universal qualities that penetrate your physical body. It contains two types of energetic vehicles—energy bodies and sheaths. In addition to energetic vehicles, your energy field contains resource fields. Resource fields provide the energy and consciousness that nourish your energetic vehicles and your subtle energy system.

Your subtle energy system includes the chakras and chakra fields, meridians, auras, and minor energy centers scattered through your subtle energy field.

In the same way that an electrical grid provides energy to homes and businesses, the organs of your subtle energy system transmit and transmute all the prana your physical body and your energetic vehicles need to function healthfully.

In the pages that follow, we will look more deeply at the organs of your subtle energy system. The chakras, chakra fields, and minor energy centers will get our particular attention because it's by skillfully using them, in chakra healing, that you will find energetic solutions for the most common problems that disrupt your life and relationships. These are problems that have as their foundation blockages in your energy field.

Normally, blockages in your subtle energy field are created when a concentration of subtle energy with individual qualities prevents prana (energy with universal qualities) from radiating freely through a chakra or minor energy center. The concentration of energy we're talking about can look like a wave or small pool of dense energy that is active and can move, especially when you pay attention to it. Because of its density and its ability to move, it can block prana the same way dirt can block the free flow of clean air through an air filter.

It's these blockages that cause attachments as well as self-limiting and destructive patterns. Many of these blockages have been with you for lifetimes since you carry the energy that supports them in your energy field from one incarnation to the next.

The chakras, chakra fields, and minor energy centers are primarily responsible for regulating energetic activities in the non-physical universe. These activities include many interactions that people mistakenly believe take place exclusively on the physical plane. Empathy, motivation, and enthusiasm as well as human love and intimacy are examples of energetic interactions regulated by the chakras, chakra fields, and energy centers in the hands and feet.

This means that the condition of your energy system can have an influence on your ability to feel and express your emotions and feelings. Unfortunately, it also means that when there are blockages in your subtle energy system, you will find that your ability to interact with your environment and with other people will be blocked.

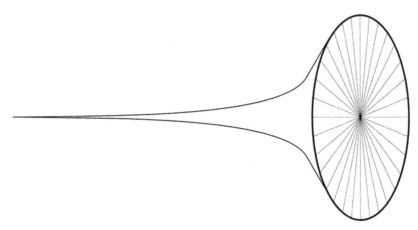

*Figure 6: The Chakra Gate*

## The Chakras

The word *chakra* comes from Sanskrit and means "wheel." There are two distinct parts of a chakra—the chakra gate and the chakra field. For people with the ability to see subtle energy fields, a chakra gate will look like a brightly colored disk that spins rapidly at the end of what looks like a long axle or stalk. The wheel portion of the chakra gate is about three inches (about eight centimeters) in diameter and perpetually moves or spins around a central axis. Emerging from the center of the disk are what appear to be spokes.

The main function of the chakra gate is to provide the subtle energy field and physical body with prana. Although chakra gates have additional functions, the principle part of a chakra is the vast reservoir of prana, which we call the chakra field. The chakra field is connected to the chakra gate. And the healthier the chakra field, the more prana will be distributed by the chakra gate to your energy field and physical body.

## Functions of the Chakras

Chakra gates and their fields are able to perform several important functions besides providing your subtle energy field and physical body with prana. They link all human beings to Universal Consciousness, the singularity from which everything in the physical and non-physical universe emerged.

They transmute prana from one pitch (or frequency) to another. The transmutation of prana takes place automatically whenever an energy body, sheath, or your physical body is in an energy-deficient condition.

Chakras also help balance the forces of polarity and gender in your energy field by permitting prana to move through your subtle energy system in four general directions, up the back, down the front, forward from the back to the front, and backward from the front to the back.

Maintaining a healthy balance between the forces of polarity and gender by distributing prana from one part of your subtle energy system to another will empower you and enhance your ability to express yourself fully.

## The Thirteen Chakras in Body Space

There are 146 chakras within the human energy system. The thirteen most important chakras are located within your body space: the seven traditional chakras located along the spine and in the head, two etheric chakras, two physical chakras, and two physical-material chakras. Below is a short list of the individual activities controlled by the thirteen chakras in your body space and the functions of mind, soul, and body they regulate.

### First Chakra

Security, self-confidence, body image, connection to the earth and its creatures. If the chakra is blocked, your relationship to your physical body will be disrupted.

### Second Chakra

Vitality, gender identity (masculinity or femininity), creativity. If the chakra is blocked, you will experience anger.

### Third Chakra

Belonging, contentment, intimacy, friendship, status, and psychic well-being. If the chakra is blocked, you will experience fear.

### Fourth Chakra

Self-awareness, personal rights (this includes the right to control your physical body, to express your feelings and emotions—and to share what you know). If the chakra is blocked, you will experience pain.

### Fifth Chakra

Self-expression, enjoyment, perseverance, and personal integrity. If the chakra is blocked, your experience of joy will be disrupted.

### Sixth Chakra

Awareness, memory, intuition, reasoning, and rational, deductive thought. If the chakra is blocked, you will experience a disruption in inductive and deduction reasoning and intuition.

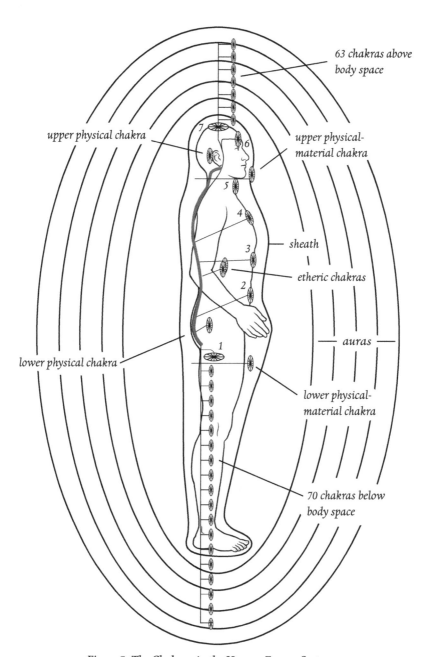

*Figure 7: The Chakras & the Human Energy System*

### Seventh Chakra

Transcendental consciousness. If the chakra is blocked, your experience of transcendence will also be blocked.

### Etheric Chakras

Regulate feelings. There are hundreds of authentic feelings that emerge from the etheric chakras ranging from comfort and satisfaction to fatigue and enthusiasm. If the chakras are blocked, your access to feelings and your ability to express them will be blocked.

### Physical Chakras

Responsible for regulating physical pleasure, particularly sexual pleasure. When the physical chakras are blocked, you will feel locked outside of yourself, on the physical level, with a corresponding loss of sensitivity to other people.

### Physical-Material Chakras

Responsible for grounding you in the physical-material world. Being grounded allows you to experience your physical body and your physical environment without disruption. When the physical-material chakras are blocked, strength and stamina will be disrupted. So will the production of pleasure producing compounds in the brain.

---

## Exercises: Sensing the Chakras in Body Space

In our work, we've found that even when people have learned something about the structure and function of the chakras, they are unable to sense them. This is unfortunate because there are simple ways to sense the chakras. One way is to use the power of running water to stimulate them.

This is easy to do in the shower. Simply direct the stream of water from the shower to the front of your first chakra, which extends from the base of your spine to a point three inches (about eight centimeters) below it. Continue until you feel a vibration emerging from the point where the chakra gate is located. Take a moment to enjoy the resonance—then move the showerhead to the second chakra, four finger widths below the navel. After a few moments, you will feel the unique vibration of the second chakra. Continue to use the water, emerging from the nozzle, to stimulate your third through seventh chakras, then your etheric, physical, and physical-material chakras. You can see the position of the chakras by consulting Figure 7.

Once you're finished stimulating your chakras, take about ten minutes to enjoy their enhanced resonance, which will continue, even after you've finished stimulating them.

Another way to sense the chakras in your body space is to rub your hands together and then place the palm of your positive hand, right hand if you're right-handed, left hand if you're left-handed, about three inches (about eight centimeters) in front of each chakra gate.

Rubbing your hands together polarizes them slightly, making it easier for you to sense the resonance of each chakra consciously. If you begin by rubbing your hands together and then place your positive hand above your first chakra gate, your palm will register its unique resonance.

To continue the process, remove your hand. Rub your hands together again and then place the palm of your positive hand in front of the second chakra gate, four finger widths below your navel. Your palm will register a slightly higher resonance than your first chakra. Continue in the same way by rubbing your palms together and then experiencing the unique resonance of the third, fourth, fifth, sixth and seventh chakras.

Once you've experienced the resonance of the seven traditional chakras, use the same technique to sense the resonance of your etheric, physical, and physical-material chakras.

After you've finished stimulating all thirteen chakras, take a few minutes to enjoy the effects you experience, emotionally, mentally and spiritually.

---

## Exercise: Activating a Chakra

Now that you can sense the chakras in your body space, you can take the next step in chakra healing by activating one of your chakras. You will learn the technique by activating your heart chakra. Then you can use the same technique to activate the other twelve chakras in your body space.

To activate your heart chakra, find a comfortable position with your back straight. Close your eyes and breathe deeply through your nose for two to three minutes. Then count backward from five to one and from ten to one. Use the Standard Method to relax and center yourself in your authentic mind (go to chapter 2).

When you're ready to continue, assert, *"It's my intent to activate my heart chakra."* Once you've activated your heart chakra, you'll feel a glowing sensation along with a heightened sense of well-being. You can enhance these effects by asserting, *"It's my intent to turn my organs of perception inward on the level of my heart chakra."* By turning your organs of perception inward, you'll become even more conscious of the shift that has taken place now that your heart chakra is active. Remain centered in your authentic mind with your attention focused on your heart chakra for fifteen minutes.

After fifteen minutes, you can return to normal consciousness by counting from one to five. When you reach the number five, open your eyes. You will feel wide-awake, perfectly relaxed, and better than you did before. Repeat as needed.

## Exercise: Centering Yourself in a Chakra Field

After you've activated your heart chakra, the next step in chakra healing is to center yourself in the corresponding chakra field. By centering yourself in the chakra field, your awareness will emerge directly from the reservoir of prana that animates you—and the heart of every radiant woman.

To center yourself in your heart chakra field, find a comfortable position with your back straight. Close your eyes and breathe deeply through your nose for two to three minutes. Count backward from five to one and from ten to one. Then use the Standard Method to relax and to center yourself in your authentic mind. When you're ready to continue, assert, *"It's my intent to activate my heart chakra."* Take a few moments to enjoy the effects. Then assert, *"It's my intent to center myself in my heart chakra field."* You can enhance the effects by turning your organs of perception inward. To do that, assert, *"It's my intent to turn my organs of perception inward on the level of my heart chakra field."* Remain centered in your heart chakra field for fifteen minutes. After fifteen minutes, you can return to normal consciousness by counting from one to five. When you reach the number five, open your eyes. You will feel wide-awake, perfectly relaxed, and better than you did before. Repeat as needed.

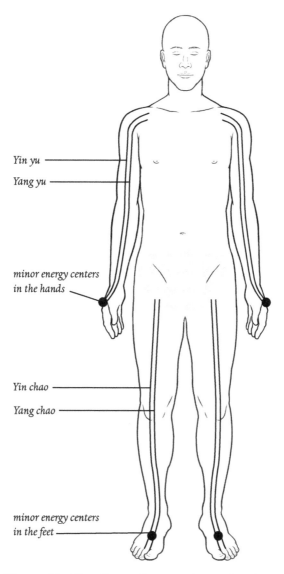

*Figure 8: The Minor Energy Centers in the Hands and Feet*

## Minor Energy Centers & Meridians

Now that you can activate your heart chakra and center yourself in your heart chakra field, you're ready to activate the minor energy centers in your hands and feet.

Everyone has four minor energy centers, one in each hand and one in each foot. These energy centers complement the functions of the chakras and have an important influence on your health and your ability to express your feminine power freely.

Minor energy centers shouldn't be confused with the chakras. Chakras are vortices through which prana enters the human energy field. Minor energy centers are centers of activity created by the functional interaction of two major meridians, one masculine and one feminine.

## Meridians

Meridians are streams of prana that have two important functions: They connect the chakras and minor energy centers, scattered throughout your energy system, to one another. And they transmit prana to the parts of the human energy field where it's needed most. By transmitting prana, the meridians keep the human energy system in balance and functioning healthfully.

Our knowledge of meridians comes from Asia. In fact, the word meridian is co-related to the Chinese word *jingxian*. The Chinese term *jingxian* corresponds to the Sanskrit word *nadi*.

Although meridians are often compared to the veins and arteries in the human circulatory system, structurally they more closely resemble currents of water and/or air found in the earth's oceans and atmosphere. While the veins and arteries have a precise structure (they are essentially long elastic tubes) with a consistent shape and carrying capacity, in contrast, meridians are streams of prana whose size and shape are regulated by the quantity of prana they carry.

If the minor energy centers are functioning healthfully, prana will radiate through the meridians in your arms and legs, and then through the minor energy centers in your hands and feet. The prana emerging from the minor energy centers in your hands will help you manifest your power, creativity and radiance freely. Those in your feet will provide you with the prana you need to move forward and make progress in the world.

---

## Exercise: Activating the Minor Energy Centers in Your Hands

The two exercises that follow are designed to activate the minor energy centers in your hands and feet. You will activate the minor energy centers in your hands first. Afterward you will activate the minor energy centers in your feet.

To begin, find a comfortable position with your back straight. Breathe deeply through your nose for two to three minutes. Then count backward from five to one and from ten to one. Use the Standard Method to relax your muscles and to center yourself in your authentic mind. Then assert, *"It's my intent to activate the energy center in my right palm."* Continue by asserting, *"It's my intent to activate the energy center in my left palm."* Once your energy centers in your hands are active, take fifteen minutes to enjoy the enhanced flow of prana radiating through them.

After fifteen minutes, count from one to five. When you reach the number five, open your eyes. You will feel wide-awake, perfectly relaxed, and better than you did before. Repeat as needed.

---

## Exercise: Activating the Minor Energy Centers in Your Feet

To begin, find a comfortable position with your back straight. Breathe deeply through your nose for two to three minutes. Then count backward from five to one and from ten to one. Use the Standard Method to relax your muscles and to center yourself in your authentic mind. Then assert, *"It's my intent to activate the energy center in my right sole."* Continue by asserting, *"It's my intent to activate the energy center in my left sole."* Once your energy centers in your feet are active, take fifteen minutes to enjoy the enhanced flow of prana radiating through them. After fifteen minutes, count from one to five. When you reach the number five, open your eyes. You will feel wide-awake, perfectly relaxed, and better than you did before. Repeat as needed.

## Getting More of What a Woman Needs

Our thoughts, emotions, and feelings are constantly interacting with the organs of the energy system and the prana radiating through it. That means if you hold on to restrictive beliefs and self-limiting patterns, prana can be blocked, physical organs can be weakened, and emotions and awareness can be disrupted. Taken together, these symptoms can create lifelong issues that will affect your relationships, work, and well-being.

## Laura's Story

Laura's story illustrates how blockages in the human energy system can influence a woman's well-being and relationships.

When Laura consulted us, she'd been working for several years as a project manager for a large German corporation. She had been able to function effectively in her profession because she was intellectually astute and took pains to control every aspect of her work.

Unfortunately, Laura hadn't recognized that her need to control every aspect of her work and environment was a result of her inability to feel herself or other people: in effect, she lacked empathy. After checking her energy field, we discovered that an energy blockage by her first chakra had blocked the flow of prana. This in turn had disrupted both her empathy and intuition.

Later in the session, Laura explained that she lived with her third husband, but that her relationship wasn't working because she found it impossible to trust men. We looked for the cause of her marital problems and discovered that she had a third chakra blockage caused by a sexual trauma she'd experienced as a teenager.

A more comprehensive analysis of her energy field at the end of her second session revealed that her other symptoms, which included an insensitivity to her body, an inability to achieve orgasm except by auto-stimulation, compulsive cleanliness, and recurrent sleep problems, stemmed from blockages in her second through sixth chakras.

In her third session, we began to teach her the skills of chakra healing, which included simple techniques to activate her chakras, center herself in her chakra fields, and fill her chakra fields with prana. The process, which Laura embraced enthusiastically, had an immediate effect. Within days, she began to empathize with her husband. This took pressure off the relationship. A short time later, her feelings began to re-emerge and she was able to feel her body again. Laura continues to practice the techniques of chakra healing and we continue to monitor her progress.

Laura's experience is not unique. Many women who've suffered from energy blockages and disruptions to their subtle energy field have learned to overcome the effects by using the techniques of chakra healing. If they can do it, so can you!

In the pages that follow, we've listed some of the most common issues afflicting women, which have their foundation in energetic blockages that restrict the flow of prana through a woman's subtle energy field. Along with a description of the issue, we've provided a series of exercises derived from chakra healing that can be used to heal them.

The issues we've listed are complex and often defy conventional cures. However, it's important to recognize that at the root of all physical and psychological issues are energetic issues that can only be solved by working directly on the human energy field.

## Exercise: Issue—Body Image Problems

Body image problems are directly related to basic insecurity. Basic insecurity afflicts a woman when her first chakra has been blocked and she doesn't have access to the frequencies of prana that make her feel secure in her subtle energy field and physical body.

A woman's first chakra can be blocked if her parents don't want her, if they don't want a girl, or if a girl has had her self-esteem disrupted by projections of energy with individual qualities from family members, friends, and people in authority. It can also be blocked if a woman remains attached to past life relationships.

It's not well known, but people who are attached to fields of energy with individual qualities can project that energy at other people. The energy projected can disrupt the energy field of the person targeted (as well as the person projecting it) and can contribute to energetic and physical disease.

A woman's first chakra can also be blocked if she has been sexually abused, especially if the perpetrator was in a position of authority.

*Solution*

To overcome body image problems at their source, you will activate your first chakra and center yourself in your first chakra field. Then you will use your intent to fill your first chakra field with prana.

To begin, find a comfortable position with your back straight. Breathe deeply through your nose for two to three minutes. Then count backward from five to one and from ten to one. Use the Standard Method to relax your muscles and to center yourself in your authentic mind. Then assert, *"It's my intent to activate my first chakra."* Your energy system knows exactly what to do next. So, don't help the process along by working too hard. Don't visualize anything or focus on your breathing. A relaxed and flexible mind is your greatest asset in energy work and healing. After you've activated your first chakra, assert, *"It's my intent to center myself in my first chakra field."* To complete the process, assert, *"It's my intent to fill my first chakra field with prana."* Don't do anything after that. Prana will fill the first chakra field without your conscious intervention.

Take fifteen minutes to enjoy the process. During that time, stay centered and remember to be here now. Let thoughts and feelings come and go while the process guides you into a deeper and richer experience. Then return to normal consciousness by counting from one to five. When you reach the number five, open your eyes. You will feel wide-awake, perfectly relaxed, and better than you did before. Practice the technique every day for two weeks and you will notice a dramatic shift in your relationship to your body.

## Exercise: Issue—Feeling Like a Sexual Object

If your environment as a child was sexualized by an adult man, if you were programmed to be your father's surrogate wife or his little princess, if you were conditioned as a child to believe that your value depended on whether you are sexually attractive to a man, or if you continuously compete with other women to prove you are sexually dominant, then you can use your second chakra and your fifth chakra to overcome these issues.

Your second chakra regulates sexual joy, sensuality, and gender orientation. Your fifth chakra regulates self-expression and unconditional joy. By enhancing the functions of these two chakras, you can disconnect yourself from the pattern that connects pleasure and joy to the sexual needs of men. In this way you will regain your sense of self-worth without giving up pleasure, joy, or your natural sexual power.

### Solution

To overcome this issue, you will activate your second chakra and center yourself in your second chakra field. Then you will fill your second chakra field with prana. Next, you will activate your fifth chakra and center yourself in your fifth chakra field. Then you will fill your fifth chakra field with prana.

To begin, find a comfortable position with your back straight. Breathe deeply through your nose for two to three minutes. Then count backward from five to one and from ten to one. Use the Standard Method to relax your muscles and to center yourself in your authentic mind. Then assert, *"It's my intent to activate my second chakra."* Continue by asserting, *"It's my intent to center myself in my second chakra field."* Take a few moments to enjoy the shift. Then assert, *"It's my intent to fill my second chakra field with prana."* After you've filled your second chakra field with prana, assert, *"It's my intent to activate my fifth chakra."* Then assert, *"It's my intent to center myself in my fifth chakra field."* Take a few moments to enjoy the shift; then assert, *"It's my intent to fill my fifth chakra field with prana."*

Take fifteen minutes to enjoy the effects. Then return to normal consciousness by counting from one to five. When you reach the number five, open your eyes. You will feel wide-awake, perfectly relaxed, and better than you did before. Practice the technique every day for two weeks and you will notice a dramatic shift in the amount of joy you experience in your body, soul, and spirit.

## Exercise: Issue—Lack of Sexual Excitement

Many women experience a lack of sexual excitement in their lives, especially when they've been in long-term relationships with a partner who can't share intimacy or celebrate the universal qualities of the feminine with them.

Such people have the tendency to project distorted energy into their partner's energy field to control their sexual expression and create a comfortable environment for themselves. Projections of distorted energy can block the flow of prana through a woman's subtle energy field and interfere with her ability to feel sexual excitement and/or express it freely.

### Solution

To overcome this issue, you will activate your heart chakra and center yourself in your heart chakra field. Then you will activate your first and second chakra, center yourself in both chakra fields, and fill your first and second chakra fields with prana.

To begin, find a comfortable position with your back straight. Breathe deeply through your nose for two to three minutes. Then count backward from five to one and from ten to one. Use the Standard Method to relax your muscles and to center yourself in your authentic mind. Then assert, *"It's my intent to activate my heart chakra."* Continue by asserting, *"It's my intent to center myself in my heart chakra field."* Take a few moments to enjoy the shift. Then assert, *"It's my intent to activate my first chakra."* After you've activated your first chakra, assert, *"It's my intent to center myself in my first chakra field."* Continue by asserting, *"It's my intent to fill my first chakra field with prana."* Take a few moments to enjoy the shift. Then assert, *"It's my intent to activate my second chakra."* Continue by asserting, *"It's my intent to center myself in my second chakra field."* Finally, assert, *"It's my intent to fill my second chakra field with prana."*

Take fifteen minutes to enjoy the effects. Then return to normal consciousness by counting from one to five. When you reach the number five, open your eyes. You will feel wide-awake, perfectly relaxed, and better than you did before. Practice the technique every day for two weeks and you will notice a dramatic shift in your level of sexual excitement.

## Exercise: Issue—Blocked Receptivity

Many women have problems being open and receptive to the men they love. That's because it's possible for a woman to love an individual man and have negative feelings about male power and its abuse. If a woman holds on to negative feelings about male power, it can interfere with her relationship with her male partner—even if he's receptive to the qualities of the universal feminine. That's because holding on to negative feelings about male power can disrupt a woman's natural polarity. It does that by blocking her ability to assert energy from her heart and to receive energy by her pelvis.

By receptive, we don't mean submissive. Receptivity is the ability to accept universal masculine qualities while sharing an intimate relationship with a man. Intimacy is the essential ingredient in all successful relationships. Without it, a woman is left feeling lonely and bereft of a deep connection to the man she loves.

### Solution

To become more receptive and achieve intimacy with your partner, you will activate your heart chakra and center yourself in your heart chakra field. Then you will activate your second chakra and center yourself in your second chakra field. Once you're centered in your chakra fields, you will activate the minor energy centers in your palms.

To begin, find a comfortable position with your back straight. Breathe deeply through your nose for two to three minutes. Then count backward from five to one and from ten to one. Use the Standard Method to relax and to center yourself in your authentic mind. Then assert, *"It's my intent to activate my heart chakra."* Continue by asserting, *"It's my intent to center myself in my heart chakra field."* Take a few moments to enjoy the shift. Then assert, *"It's my intent to activate my second chakra."* Continue by asserting, *"It's my intent to center myself in my second chakra field."*

After you've centered yourself in your second chakra field, assert, *"It's my intent to activate my minor energy center in my right hand."* Next, assert, *"It's my intent to activate the minor energy center in my left hand."*

Take fifteen minutes to enjoy the effects. Then return to normal consciousness by counting from one to five. When you reach the number five, open your eyes. You will feel wide-awake, perfectly relaxed, and better than you did before. Practice the technique every day for two weeks and you will notice a dramatic shift in your receptivity and your ability to experience intimacy with your partner.

---

### Exercise: Issue—Lack of Self-Esteem

Self-esteem is so obvious to people who have it that its importance is rarely appreciated by them. But for those people who lack self-esteem, existence can be a constant struggle. Fortunately, anybody who lacks self-esteem can use their subtle energy system to free themselves from this pattern once and for all.

*Solution*

In our work, we've learned that self-esteem is directly connected to two things, self-confidence and inner joy. To increase your self-confidence and joy, you will activate your first, third, and fifth chakras and center yourself in their corresponding chakra fields. Then you will fill all three fields with prana.

To begin, breathe deeply through your nose for two to three minutes. Then count backward from five to one and from ten to one. Use the Standard Method to relax and to center yourself in your authentic mind. Then assert, *"It's my intent to activate my first chakra."* Continue by asserting, *"It's my intent to center myself in my first chakra field."* Next, assert, *"It's my intent to fill my first chakra field with prana."* Take a few moments to enjoy the shift; then assert, *"It's my intent to activate my third chakra."* Continue by asserting, *"It's my intent to center myself in my third chakra field."* Next, assert, *"It's my intent to fill my third chakra field with prana."* Take a few moments to enjoy the shift. Then assert, *"It's my intent to activate my fifth chakra."* Continue by asserting, *"It's my intent to center myself in my fifth chakra field."* To complete the process, assert, *"It's my intent to fill my fifth chakra field with prana."* Enjoy the effects for fifteen minutes. Then return to normal consciousness by counting from one to five. When you reach the number five, open your eyes. You will feel wide-awake and perfectly relaxed.

Practice the technique every day for two weeks and you will experience a dramatic shift in your self-esteem and your ability to radiate power, creativity, and radiance freely.

---

### Exercise: Issue—Blaming Men for Everything

It's easy to blame men for everything that has gone wrong in your life. But blame never liberated any woman from male oppression. In fact, blame can cause a host of secondary problems that can prevent a woman from enjoying the universal qualities of the feminine. It's best to drop the blame game and use the techniques of chakra healing to liberate yourself from its effects.

#### Solution

To stop blaming men for everything, you will activate your first and third chakras and center yourself in your first and third chakra fields. Then you will activate your energy centers in your feet. It's the energy in your feet that will enable you to move forward and make progress in the world. And it's by activating your first and third chakras, and then centering yourself in the corresponding chakra fields, that will enable you to feel secure enough to stop blaming men.

To begin, breathe deeply through your nose for two to three minutes. Then count backward from five to one and from ten to one. Use the Standard Method to relax your muscles and to center yourself in your authentic mind. Then assert, *"It's my intent to activate my first chakra."* Continue by asserting, *"It's my intent to center myself in my first chakra field."* Next, assert, *"It's my intent to activate my third chakra."* Continue by asserting, *"It's my intent to center myself in my third chakra field."* Take a few moments to enjoy the shift; then assert, *"It's my intent to activate my energy center in my right sole."* Continue by asserting, *"It's my intent to activate the energy center in my left sole."* Enjoy the effects for fifteen minutes.

Then return to normal consciousness by counting from one to five. When you reach the number five, open your eyes. You will feel wide-awake and perfectly relaxed. By practicing the technique every day for two weeks, you will be able to pursue your personal goals without the blame game getting in your way.

## Exercise: Issue—Lack of Vitality or Motivation

A disruption in polarity can block the flow of prana through a woman's subtle energy field. This in turn can disrupt vitality and motivation and can lead eventually to chronic fatigue or even worse, burnout. Women are particularly susceptible to chronic fatigue and burnout because they invest more of themselves in their relationships.

### Solution

To overcome the underlying problems that disrupt vitality and motivation, you will activate your second chakra, center yourself in your second chakra field, and fill your second chakra field with prana. Then you will do the same with your lower physical-material chakra and your upper physical-material chakra.

To begin, breathe deeply through your nose for two of three minutes. Count backward from five to one and from ten to one. Use the Standard Method to relax your muscles and to center yourself in your authentic mind. Then assert, *"It's my intent to activate my second chakra."* Continue by asserting, *"It's my intent to center myself in my second chakra field."* Then assert, *"It's my intent to fill my second chakra field with prana."* Take a moment to enjoy the shift. Then assert, *"It's my intent to activate my lower physical-material chakra."* Continue by asserting, *"It's my intent to center myself in my lower physical-material chakra field."* Next, assert, *"It's my intent to fill my lower physical-material chakra field with prana."* Take a moment to enjoy the shift. Then assert, *"It's my intent to activate my upper physical-material chakra."* Continue by asserting, *"It's my intent to center myself in my upper physical-material chakra field."* Then assert, *"It's my intent to fill my upper physical-material chakra field with prana."* Enjoy the effects for fifteen minutes.

Then return to normal consciousness by counting from one to five. When you reach the number five, open your eyes. You will feel wide-awake and perfectly relaxed. Practice the technique every day for two weeks and you will notice an increase in your vitality and motivation.

# Exercise: Issue—
## Holding On to Negative Attachments

Suffering is caused by attachment to restrictive beliefs and self-limiting patterns. If you are unable to overcome your attachments, suffering can become a day-to-day ordeal that can disrupt motivation and self-esteem and interfere with intimate relationships. Although giving up attachments is a lifelong process, you can use your chakras, and the prana emerging from them, to weaken your attachments, so that you can experience more pleasure, love, intimacy, and joy in your life and relationships now.

### Solution

To overcome negative attachments, you will begin a thirteen-day process of chakra healing. On each day, you will activate a chakra, center yourself in the corresponding chakra field, and then fill the chakra field with prana. To view the location of the thirteen chakras in body space, see figure 7.

On day one, you will activate your first chakra and center yourself in your first chakra field. Then you will fill the first chakra field with prana. On the next twelve days, you will continue in the same way by working on the remaining twelve chakras in this order: second through seventh traditional chakras, lower and upper etheric chakras, lower and upper physical chakras, and finally the lower and upper physical-material chakras.

To begin, breathe deeply through your nose for two or three minutes. Then count backward from five to one and from ten to one. Use the Standard Method to relax your muscles and to center yourself in your authentic mind. Then assert, *"It's my intent to activate my first chakra."* Continue by asserting, *"It's my intent to center myself in my first chakra field."* Once you're centered in the first chakra field, assert, *"It's my intent to fill my first chakra field with prana."* Take ten minutes to enjoy the effects.

Then count from one to five. When you reach the number five, open your eyes. You will feel wide-awake and perfectly relaxed. By activating the first chakra, centering yourself in the first chakra field, and then filling the first chakra field with prana, you will weaken the attachments that interfere with the sensations and activities that your first chakra supports. You can continue to overcome attachments that have limited you by working your second through thirteenth chakras in your body space for twelve more days. Repeat as needed.

## Summary

In this chapter, you learned how to distinguish the difference between energy with universal qualities and energy with individual qualities, and you learned how to use the organs of your energy system to perform chakra healing. By using the skills you developed in this chapter, you can heal self-limiting and destructive patterns that have prevented you from sharing your energy and consciousness freely.

In the next chapter, you will take the next step in the process of healing by learning how karmic baggage, a form of energy with individual qualities, can disrupt the functions of your subtle energy field. Then you will learn to use your intent, mental attention, and bliss, the most powerful force available to you, to heal karmic wounds that have their foundation in karmic baggage. You will also learn to use your healing skills along with your functions of mind to overcome the influence of restrictive beliefs that have prevented you from accessing all the power, creativity, and radiance available to you.

## FOUR

# Healing Karmic Wounds

Every woman alive today lives with the legacy of her past life activities in her subtle energy field in the form of karmic baggage. Overcoming karmic baggage and the wounds it supports is an essential part of healing your body, soul, and spirit.

Karmic baggage is composed of dense energy with individual qualities. Even a small amount of karmic baggage can influence the flow of prana through your energy field and create energetic blockages and self-limiting patterns that disrupt your ability to be yourself and achieve your goals. The blockages and patterns created by karmic baggage can also influence your belief system by providing energetic support to restrictive beliefs that you've integrated into your personality. Indeed, it's the presence of karmic baggage that explains why it can be so difficult to overcome restrictive beliefs or change how you feel about yourself and other people.

## What is Karmic Baggage?

To get a sense of what karmic baggage is and how it can disrupt your life and relationships, you must first know what karma is and how it functions. The ancient Sanskrit word *karma* comes from the root *kri*, "to act," and it signifies an activity or action.

In the West, karma has been defined as "the cumulative effect of action." In a limited way, this is true, though the great religions of the East go beyond this definition by describing karma in terms of both its structure and function.

Jainism, an ancient religion of India which stresses aestheticism, non-violence, and reverence for life, views karma—and by extension karmic baggage—as a subtle substance that accumulates in the human energy field.

According to this ancient religion, karmic baggage obscures comprehension and awareness; it produces counterfeit sensations, feelings, and emotions; it veils the truth; it creates self-limiting patterns; it determines status and therefore psychic well-being; and it disrupts personal power.

It should be clear by now that karmic baggage is far more complex than the abstract principle that guarantees that you will reap what you sow. Karmic baggage is a force of nature, which manifests will and intent and connects the effects of actions, on all interpenetrating worlds and dimensions, to their causes.

This means that karmic baggage functions a lot like gravity. Like gravity, the polarity karma creates between the cause and its effect can attract you to fields of distorted energy in people, places, and things and then attach you to it. Once you've become attached to a field of energy with individual qualities, a polar relationship is created which facilitates a transfer of distorted energy from the distorted field of energy to your subtle energy field. This explains how you can accumulate karmic baggage in your energy field. The more attachments you have, the more polarized your subtle energy field will become. And the more polarized your subtle energy field becomes, the more likely it will be for distorted energy to become trapped in it. If this process is allowed to continue unchecked, you can collect layers of karmic baggage that will fill large parts of your subtle energy field. In time, this karmic baggage will create blockages in your energy field that will make it difficult for you to engage in the normal activities of life, or in intimate relationships with other people.

When you've accumulated enough karmic baggage on the level of soul (intellect, emotion, and feeling) the attachments you create will make it difficult for you to feel your emotions or to express them freely. They will also disrupt your awareness, creativity, and your normal balance of inductive and deductive reasoning.

In time, you can find yourself trapped in the internal dialogue (the incessant chatter of the individual mind and ego) and reactive to fields or energy with individual qualities. When that happens, you may feel like your mind has become foggy or is racing out of control.

When you've accumulated enough karmic baggage on the level of spirit, you will find it difficult to go inward and experience the inner peace and bliss that normally emerges when you have access to the inner self (your source of bliss). This in turn will prevent you from recognizing and following your dharma.

Your spirit can be thought of as the universal aspect of mind that experiences intimacy with other living beings. It's from deep within your spirit that your intuition, insight, and discernment emerge.

Your dharma is your purpose as well as your individual path of self-healing and self-realization. Purpose includes the work you perform and the impact you will have on other people. It's by following your dharma that you will learn who you are and what you are capable of achieving in this life. The universe will support you when you follow your personal dharma by removing obstacles and by giving you what you need to overcome life's challenges.

To follow dharma, you must engage exclusively in activities that are motivated by your authentic mind. It's these activities that will promote the flow of prana through your subtle energy system, keep you centered in your authentic mind, and centered in the universal qualities of the feminine.

It's attachments created by karmic baggage, on the spiritual level, that will keep you busy with activities which lead nowhere and which merely serve to perpetuate old karmic patterns. This fruitless merry-go-round is ultimately self-defeating and antagonistic to self-awareness and freedom of self-expression. "Living in a spiritual desert" is a phrase often used to describe such a condition.

For a woman to heal her soul and spirit, she must overcome the power of the karmic baggage in her energy field and consistently put her faith in what is most real, the universal qualities of the feminine that emerge through her authentic mind. It may seem a Promethean task to overcome your karmic heritage. But the truth is many women have done it. And so can you. With that in mind, we've included an exercise that you can use to release karmic baggage and permanently free yourself from its limitations.

## Say Good-bye to Karmic Baggage

All the tools you need to release karmic baggage are contained in your subtle energy field. But they emerge into your conscious awareness through your authentic mind. The tools we're referring to include your intent, your mental attention, and transcendental consciousness in the form of bliss. By combining these three tools in the appropriate way, you will be able to locate concentrations of karmic baggage in your subtle energy field, discern their qualities, and then release them permanently.

### Your Intent

Your intent is a function of your authentic mind that is active on all worlds and dimensions of the physical and non-physical universe. In the exercise that follows, you will use your intent to program your mental attention to locate the particular concentration of karmic baggage, in your energy field, you wish to release. You can use your intent to program your mental attention to locate a concentration of karmic baggage that is responsible for a physical ailment, a blockage in your energy field, a self-limiting pattern, and/or a negative and self-destructive attitude, emotion, and feeling. After you've used your intent to program your mental attention, you will use it in conjunction with bliss to release the karmic baggage you've located.

### Your Mental Attention

Your mental attention functions simultaneously on all worlds and dimensions in both the physical and non-physical universe. With the intent as a guide, your mental attention can locate a concentration of karmic baggage and provide you with the information you need to release it. This information can include the concentration's size, shape, density, polarity, and level of activity.

### Orgasmic Bliss

Orgasmic bliss is the most powerful force in the universe. Every human being is in bliss, although most people are unaware of it. According to the tantrics, orgasmic bliss is an enduring condition, deep inside your energy field, created through the union of consciousness (Shiva) and energy (Shakti). The merging of consciousness and energy with universal qualities provides you with a constant flow of power that can release even the densest concentrations of karmic baggage.

However, to use orgasmic bliss to release karmic baggage, you must bring it into your conscious awareness and keep it there during the healing process. That's because you must radiate bliss consciously to permanently release the karmic baggage that your intent has programmed your mental attention to locate.

To bring bliss into your conscious awareness, you will learn to perform a mudra specifically designed for that purpose. That mudra is called the Orgasmic Bliss Mudra.

It's important to note that bliss is not a form of feminine energy. Rather, it is the highest form of consciousness available to human beings.

---

## Exercise: The Orgasmic Bliss Mudra

To perform the Orgasmic Bliss Mudra, use the Standard Method to relax your muscles and to center yourself in your authentic mind. Then place the tip of your tongue on your upper palate and bring it straight back until it comes to rest at the point where the hard palate rolls up and becomes soft. Once the tip of your tongue is in that position, put the bottom of your feet together so that the soles are touching. Then bring your hands in front of your solar plexus and place the inside tips of your thumbs together. Continue by bringing the outside of your index fingers together from the tips to the first joint. Next, bring the outside of your middle fingers together from the first to the second joint.

The fourth and fifth fingers should be curled into your palm. Once your tongue, fingers, and feet are in position, close your eyes and breathe through your nose.

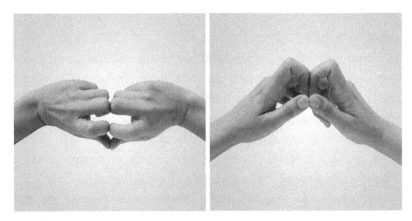

*Figure 9: The Orgasmic Bliss Mudra*

Hold the mudra for ten minutes. Then release your fingers, separate the soles of your feet, and bring your tongue back to its normal position. Next, count from one to five. When you reach the number five, open your eyes. You will be wide-awake, perfectly relaxed, and you'll feel better than you did before.

## Releasing Karmic Baggage

Now that you can perform the Orgasmic Bliss Mudra, you're ready to use your bliss along with your intent and mental attention to release a concentration of karmic baggage caught in your subtle energy field.

Your first step will be to choose what concentration of karmic baggage to release. Since karmic baggage serves as the foundation of energy blockages and self-limiting patterns as well as negative and self-destructive attitudes, emotions, and feelings, this shouldn't be difficult to do. Confusion, chaos, and ambivalence normally have a foundation in karmic baggage. So do jealousy, envy, self-doubt and contempt, rage, frustration, anxiety, emptiness, and annoyance, as well as feelings of numbness that can alienate you from your body, soul, and spirit. You could also choose a physical condition, like back pain or tooth grinding. Both have a foundation in karmic baggage.

When making your choice, it's important to remember that karmic baggage has individual qualities, which means it will feel heavier and denser than prana.

Once you've chosen an issue or pattern to work on, you will use the Standard Method to relax your muscles and to center yourself in your authentic mind. Then, you will perform the Orgasmic Bliss Mudra. After that, you will use your intent to program your mental attention to locate and release the concentration of karmic baggage you have in mind.

---

## Exercise: Releasing a Concentration of Karmic Baggage

To begin the process, find a comfortable position with your back straight. Then choose a karmically based issue, pattern, or ailment to release.

Once you've chosen an issue or pattern or ailment, close your eyes and breathe deeply through your nose for two to three minutes. Use the Standard Method to relax your muscles and to center yourself in your authentic mind. Then perform the Orgasmic Bliss Mudra. Continue to hold the mudra while you assert, *"It's my intent to create a visual screen eight feet (two-and-a-half meters) in front of me."* Once the screen has appeared, assert, *"It's my intent to visualize an image of myself on the screen."* Once the image appears, assert, *"It's my intent to locate the karmic baggage, in the image, that is responsible for my (put your issue, pattern or physical ailment here)."*

You may see or sense the concentration of karmic baggage on the screen. In either case, it will stand out from the background because it will feel denser or heavier, look darker, or put pressure on your energy field. In some cases, it may even cause physical discomfort.

Once you've located the concentration of karmic baggage, you will create a prana box that surrounds it. The size and shape of the box should closely follow the contours of the concentration of karmic baggage. To construct the box, assert, *"It's my intent to create a prana box around the karmic baggage I have in mind."* Once you can sense and/or see the box, assert,

*"It's my intent to fill the box with bliss and release the karmic baggage contained within it."* Don't do anything after that. Bliss will fill the box you've created. Since bliss is far more powerful than any form of energy with individual qualities, the karmic baggage in the box will be released permanently.

Some of you may experience a sense of relief and/or a pop. Both indicate that the karmic baggage within the box has been released and bliss has replaced it.

Once the karmic baggage has been released, release the box and the Orgasmic Bliss Mudra. Then count from one to five. When you reach the number five, open your eyes. You will feel wide-awake, perfectly relaxed, and better than you did before.

## Overcoming Restrictive Beliefs

Now that you can release karmic baggage, you can use the same skills to overcome the effect of restrictive beliefs that have their foundation in concentrations of karmic baggage.

A restrictive belief is any belief accepted as true by an institution of society that prevents people from expressing themselves freely. Restrictive beliefs restrict the flow of prana and make it difficult for people to stay centered in their energy fields. They have an inordinate effect on women because they limit a woman's power, creativity, and radiance. They do this by distorting a woman's feelings about her body and herself, and by making it difficult for a woman to create a healthy and authentic identity.

Because restrictive beliefs force women to contract energetically, they can increase self-limiting and/or destructive tendencies such as chronic insecurity, anxiety, depression, hypersensitivity, and "game playing." In extreme cases, a restrictive belief can even create obsessions, which in turn can cause anti-self and anti-social behavior.

As far back as 1955, the celebrated author e.e. cummings noted that "to be nobody but yourself in a world which is doing its best, night and day, to make you like everybody else means to fight the hardest battle which any human being can fight."

## The Fabulous Functions of Mind

To overcome the effects of restrictive beliefs that inhibit you from embracing and sharing prana freely, you must use your functions of mind. Functions of mind, like your intent, emerge from your authentic mind. They allow you to participate spontaneously in all the activities of the physical and non-physical universe and to experience the world directly without programming and restrictive beliefs getting in the way. They also provide you with the power to overcome all the limitations that restrictive beliefs have created in your life.

There are sixteen important functions of mind through which your power, creativity, and radiance emerge. You've already learned to use your "intent" to perform chakra healing and to release karmic baggage. There are fifteen others including will, desire, resistance, surrender, acceptance, knowing, choice, commitment, rejection, faith, enjoyment, destruction, creativity, empathy, and love.

## Taking the First Step

To overcome a restrictive belief, you will use your authentic functions of mind in conjunction with a positive affirmation. A positive affirmation can be defined as a statement that is objectively true. *"I am a radiant woman and have all of the universal qualities of the feminine within me"* is such a statement. It is objectively true because it cannot be modified by culture or a restrictive belief system. And it's true everywhere in all situations.

Replacing a restrictive belief with an assertion that is objectively true will have a profound effect on you. It will enhance your self-esteem and the flow of feminine energy through your energy field. And it will keep you centered in your authentic mind.

## Affirmations for the Twenty-First Century

Traditional affirmations normally used one function of mind to overcome restrictive beliefs. But in our experience, we've learned that it's more effective to use more than one authentic function of the mind to overcome a restrictive belief. There is a good reason for this: each function of mind will liberate a specific spectrum of prana that has been blocked by your attachment to a restrictive belief.

This means that by using more than one function of mind, you can more readily counteract the influence of a restrictive belief in your life—and then overcome it. *"I must be in control of every aspect of my life"* is a restrictive belief that will illustrate our point. When the restrictive belief comes up, you can counteract it by asserting, *"I have faith in and love the universal feminine, so it's not necessary for me to control every aspect of my life."* Then you can overcome it by using two additional functions of mind, "knowing" and "acceptance," to assert, *"I know and accept that I can remain open and flexible in every situation."* Positive affirmations will work best when you assert the affirmation clearly and firmly in a normal voice.

## Exercise: Using Positive Affirmations

You can use positive affirmations whenever a restrictive belief disturbs you, or as part of your meditations and regimen of energy work. To begin, make a short list of restrictive beliefs that interfere with your ability to experience your feminine power, creativity, and radiance. Leave room underneath each restrictive belief. Then decide on the appropriate affirmations and the functions of mind that you will use to release them, and write it underneath. Keep the restrictive belief in mind for a few moments. Then repeat the appropriate affirmations to yourself in words, rather than in thoughts, along with the functions of mind you've chosen to support it. Repeat the affirmations for at least five minutes, or until the restrictive belief no longer disturbs you. It's a good idea to work on one or two restrictive beliefs at a time. After they've been released, you can repeat the process, another time, with the remaining restrictive beliefs on your list.

A sample list of restrictive beliefs is provided below:

1. I need to be perfect at everything I do.
2. I have to have a thin body in order to be attractive.
3. Surrendering to an intimate relationship with a man is a sign of weakness.

4. I have to be in control of every aspect of my life.

5. It is not enough to be myself and radiate prana through my body, soul, and spirit.

6. What I do is more important than who I am.

7. The more I have the more successful I am.

8. Powerful women are too masculine.

To help guide you through the process, we've included three restrictive beliefs from the above list along with a sample of affirmations and functions of mind that you can use to release them. We suggest you use two functions of mind to counteract a restrictive belief, and then another two functions of mind to overcome it. For example, to counteract and overcome the restrictive belief that "The more I have the more successful I am," you can use faith and knowing and assert, *"I have faith and know that success is determined by being myself and expressing myself freely."* Then you can use knowing and commitment to assert, *"I know it's appropriate and I'm committed to sharing my power, creativity, and radiance through my work and relationships."*

To counteract the belief that "You have to have a thin body to be attractive," you can use acceptance and enjoyment and assert, *"I accept and enjoy the body, soul, and spirit that is the universe's gift to me."* Then you can use knowing and faith to assert, *"I know and have faith that inner beauty is a woman's greatest treasure."*

To counteract the belief that "What I do is more important than who I am," you can use desire and knowing and assert, *"I desire and know that that my success depends on being the most powerful, creative, and radiant woman I can be."* Then you can use will and desire to assert, *"It's my will and desire to become the powerful, creative, and radiant woman I'm supposed to be in this life."*

Use the affirmations that we've provided as a foundation. Then be as creative as you like. Don't be discouraged if you don't counteract and overcome a restrictive belief immediately. Continue to use affirmations along with the appropriate functions of mind regularly, and in a short time you will overcome the influence of the restrictive beliefs that have limited you.

***

## Exercise: A Regimen of Affirmations

You don't have to use positive affirmations and functions of mind solely for releasing restrictive beliefs. You can also use them to enhance your well-being. The list that follows includes positive affirmations that are objectively true, as well as one or more functions of mind that support them. You can use them whenever you have the time and the desire, will, and intent to enhance your well-being and relationships.

1. I accept and know that I have an unlimited supply of feminine energy within me.
2. I accept and know that it's my birthright to express my power, creativity, and radiance freely.
3. I have faith and accept that it's appropriate for me to make my own decisions.
4. I have faith and I know that I am stronger than my programming; I'm a radiant, powerful woman.
5. I accept and know that I am more than the sum of my parts. I am a manifestation of the universal feminine.
6. It's my desire and will to transcend the restrictive elements of my belief system.
7. It's my intent to love myself as I am and not how other people want me to be.
8. It's my desire and will to express my authentic feminine identity freely.
9. It's my intent, desire, and will to love what gives me pleasure.
10. It's my intent, desire, and will to love my body and my unique sexual identity.

## Summary

In this chapter, you learned how attachments created by karmic baggage can disrupt your relationship to your self, to the universal feminine, and to the people you love. Then you learned how to release it by using your intent, mental attention, and bliss. You also learned to use your functions of mind to overcome restrictive beliefs and replace them with life affirmations that support your power, creativity, and radiance. In the next chapter, you will learn how to create a life-affirming identity by healing your aspects of mind and by overcoming self-limiting cultural archetypes.

Aspects of mind are subtle energetic vehicles that allow you to make contact with people, places, and things in your external environment. Once you've healed your aspects of mind, you will learn how to overcome self-limiting archetypes that have blocked you and replace them with life-affirming archetypes that support your power, creativity, and radiance.

# FIVE

# Creating a Life-Affirming Identity

Without having a life-affirming identity as an anchor, a woman's spirit will remain adrift and her soul will suffer needlessly. A life-affirming identity is an essential part of the joyful life of a radiant woman. In this chapter, we will show you how you can restore and refine your identity so that it supports your relationship to the universal feminine and to your self.

A life-affirming feminine identity is one that has as its foundation self-confidence, self-esteem, and empathy for others. For a modern woman, creating a life-affirming identity is an essential part of healing her soul and spirit. Chakra healing and releasing karmic baggage are important steps in creating a life-affirming identity. However, to complete the process, you must be able to restore your aspects of mind and overcome unhealthy archetypes that have been integrated into your personality and therefore form a part of your identity.

Aspects of mind are subtle energetic vehicles that serve as the foundation of your authentic identity. Archetypes are templates or energetic holographs that determine how you see yourself, what you value, how you judge others, and whether you will follow your dharma. Some archetypes owe their existence to past life karma, which means that you've carried them with you from past lives. Others are created by early childhood programming and the acculturation process.

## Healing Aspects of Mind

The restoration of your life-affirming identity begins when you heal your aspects of mind. Aspects of mind are slightly larger than energy bodies, which means they extend a few centimeters beyond the space occupied by your physical body on the physical plane.

What differentiates aspects of mind from your other energetic vehicles is their ability to extend themselves beyond your energy field—so that they can make contact with other people and energy fields in their environment. This ability to extend and then to contract makes your aspects of mind ideal vehicles for gaining knowledge and orientating yourself in the world. It also makes the aspects of mind vulnerable to contamination by distorted fields of energy in the external environment. Adding to the problem is the fact that people can project contaminated aspects of mind at one another. When a contaminated aspect of mind makes contact with your energy field, it can become attached to your energy field along with the distorted energy that has contaminated it.

It's only by releasing unhealthy aspects of mind projected into your energy field and by decontaminating your own aspects of mind that you can establish the life-affirming identity you need to emerge as a powerful, self-contained woman.

According to the ancient texts of tantra, there are four aspects of mind. In Sanskrit, they are known as the manas, buddhi, chitta, and ahamkara.

The manas extends itself until it makes contact with an object, being, and/or energy field in the external environment, thus isolating itself so it can be studied. The manas aspect can be understood using the metaphor of looking as opposed to seeing. When looking, there is no emphasis put on anything in particular. But in seeing, that which is seen is brought into a context where it can be compared and studied. The manas doesn't look; rather it sees by putting emphasis on something in its field of vision so that it can be separated from its environment.

The buddhi analyzes and compares an object, person, and/or energy field that has been separated from its environment with what is already known. Although objects, people, and/or energy fields may vary and/or change, the buddhi remains constant. In fact, it's the buddhi's consistency that allows it to put what it has studied into a specific context so that the chitta can confer a particular value on it.

The chitta confers a value on what has been isolated by manas and analyzed by buddhi. Value depends on the condition of the human being making contact with their environment through their aspects of mind. When a woman is attached to restrictive beliefs and self-limiting archetypes, the value of something will be determined by whether it furthers physical and/or psychic well-being. When a woman has chosen to heal herself and restore her power, creativity, and radiance, the value of something will be determined by whether it enhances her relationship to her self and the universal qualities of the feminine.

Ahamkara is the decision maker and distills the information it receives from the other three aspects of mind to create and/or support a woman's view of herself and her relationships. What it receives and accepts as valid and relevant not only adds to what a woman accepts as "knowledge," it confirms experientially what she already knows about herself.

When the information supports restrictive beliefs and self-limiting archetypes, it will disrupt a woman's relationship to feminine energy and it will prevent a woman from experiencing the satisfaction that comes from knowing and following her dharma. When the decision supports the universal qualities of the feminine, it will confirm what a woman intuitively knows about herself: that she is the physical manifestation of the universal feminine.

By the time you reached puberty, it's likely that you became attached to contaminated aspects of mind projected into your energy field. Some of the most common effects are included in the list below. If you've experienced any of these effects, you can use the exercises that follow to overcome them.

## Effects of Foreign Aspects of Mind

1. You're overly reactive to the opinions of other people.
2. You feel fragile or inordinately shy in public.
3. You feel self-conscious and insecure.
4. You've become alienated from your feelings and your body.
5. You've become overly dependent on other people.
6. You find it difficult to find and/or follow your dharma.
7. You feel smothered by the needs and expectations of other people.
8. You find it difficult to express your true feelings and/or ideas.
9. You feel exhausted or drained by people at least some of the time.
10. You're constantly looking for your "self" without success.

Our list is only a sample. But if you feel trapped by any persistent issue or pattern that continuously interferes with ability to manifest a strong, life-affirming identity, or you know a person who has interfered with your ability to be yourself or to express yourself freely, then it's likely that you've become attached to one or more foreign aspects of mind.

In the exercise that follows, you will learn how to decontaminate and release a contaminated aspect of mind that has become attached to your energy field. After that, you will learn how to decontaminate one of your own aspects of mind, so that your soul and spirit are free to fulfill their authentic purpose.

## Exercise: Releasing Foreign Aspects of Mind

To decontaminate and release a foreign aspect of mind, find a comfortable position with your back straight. Choose an issue or identity problem from our list to work on. If none of them applies, choose a different issue or identity problem that you believe has disrupted your ability to manifest a strong, life-affirming identity. Keep it in mind. Then close your eyes and breathe deeply through your nose for two to three minutes. Use the Standard Method to relax your muscles and to center yourself in your authentic mind. Then perform the Orgasmic Bliss Mudra (go to chapter 4). Hold the mudra while you assert, *"It's my intent to create a visual screen eight feet (two-and-a-half meters) in front of me."* Once the screen has appeared, assert, *"It's my intent to visualize an image of myself on the screen."* Once the image appears, assert, *"It's my intent to locate the foreign aspect of mind whose energy supplies the most support to the issue I have in mind."* If it's a foreign aspect of mind it will be shaped like a flexible tube that intrudes into your body space and extends outside of your field for a significant distance. Once you've verified that it's a foreign aspect of mind by its shape, assert, *"It's my intent to surround the aspect of mind I have in mind with a prana box."* The box should be big enough for the aspect of mind to fit into it snugly. Next, assert, *"It's my intent to fill the prana box with bliss and decontaminate the aspect of mind within it."* Finally, assert, *"It's my intent that the decontaminated aspect of mind returns directly to its place of origin."*

Once the foreign aspect of mind has been decontaminated and released, release the prana box. Then release the Orgasmic Bliss Mudra. Continue by releasing the image of yourself on the screen and the visual screen itself. Then count from one to five to bring yourself out of the exercise.

Many people experience a sense of relief and greater self-confidence once a foreign aspect of mind has been decontaminated and released. Others feel a greater sense of personal integrity.

When creating a more life-affirming identity it's important to remember that it's possible for more than one aspect of mind to support an issue or identity problem. If you feel that the issue persists even after you've decontaminated and released one foreign aspect of mind, repeat the process until all foreign aspects of mind that support the issue or identity problem have been decontaminated and released.

## Exercise: Reintegrating Your Personal Aspects of Mind

To form a life-affirming identity it's important that your personal aspects of mind are free of contaminants and properly integrated into your energy field. To decontaminate and reintegrate one of your own aspects of mind, find a comfortable position with your back straight. Then close your eyes and breathe deeply through your nose for two to three minutes. Use the Standard Method to relax your muscles and to center yourself in your authentic mind. Then perform the Orgasmic Bliss Mudra (go to chapter 4). Hold the mudra while you assert, *"It's my intent to create a visual screen eight feet (two-and-a-half meters) in front of me."* Once the screen has appeared, assert, *"It's my intent to visualize an image of myself on the screen."* Once the image appears, assert, *"It's my intent to locate my most contaminated aspect of mind."*

If the aspect of mind is contaminated, it will have distortions, in the form of bulges, along its edges. And it won't be properly integrated, which means it will be tilted outside body space, or it will be lying alongside it.

Once you've verified that you've located a personal aspect of mind by its shape and position, assert, *"It's my intent to surround the aspect of mind I have in mind with a prana box."* Then assert, *"It's my intent to fill the prana box with bliss and decontaminate the aspect of mind within it."* Finally, assert, *"It's my intent to reintegrate the aspect of mind I just decontaminated."* Don't do anything after that. Just enjoy the process for ten minutes.

After ten minutes, release the prana box. Then release the Orgasmic Bliss Mudra. Continue by releasing the image of yourself on the screen and the visual screen itself. Then count from one to five to bring yourself out of the exercise.

Once you've decontaminated and reintegrated a personal aspect of mind, you will experience a sense of relief and renewed self-confidence. If you continue to decontaminate and reintegrate all your contaminated aspects of mind, it won't take long for your identity to become stronger and more life-affirming.

## Overcoming Self-Limiting Archetypes

Now that you've learned to heal your aspects of mind, you're ready to overcome self-limiting archetypes of women. A self-limiting archetype is a distorted and/or superficial image of a woman that limits a woman's power, creativity, and radiance. It does this by distorting her feelings about her body and herself, and by making it difficult for a woman to create a healthy, life-affirming identity.

You may believe that you're immune from self-limiting, cultural archetypes. But we don't have to look any further than the entertainment industries and in the religious institutions that are still playing an important part in most people's lives, to see that women continue to be portrayed in distorted and unflattering ways. The truth is that laws may have been passed that liberated women from the oppressive conditions of the past, but the self-limiting archetypes of women that pervade modern societies can still trap women in distorted, ill-fitting boxes.

There are many female archetypes. There are positive and negative archetypes in most modern societies for different types of women and the significant stages of a woman's life. But surprisingly, even the positive archetypes of modern societies can be negative in their capacity to limit a woman's natural power, creativity, and radiance.

We can see this illustrated in the difficult transition that girls must negotiate during puberty. During this critical time in a young woman's life, the lack of healthy, life-affirming archetypes that take into consideration the changes and natural demands of a young woman's body and energy field is almost shocking. Indeed, during this critical period, young women in the Western world are almost completely bereft of healthy archetypes to help them establish a strong, life-affirming identity. Instead, they are left with cultural stereotypes that don't provide them with the support they need to deal with important issues such as sex, contraception, child rearing, and marriage.

In contrast, traditional matriarchal societies provide young women with far more support and with far healthier female archetypes (Di-Maria 2011).

## Rites of Passage in Other Cultures

A good example is the Dipo tribe (Akan culture), a small ethnic group that lives in the northern part of Ghana. In Akan culture, women and girls are taught to adhere to a healthy, age-appropriate archetype that imbues young women with beauty, purity, and dignity, which protects them against corruption. The Akana believe that well-taught mothers with good traditions also raise strong girls. For this reason, there is more emphasis on the female rites of passage than on the male ones.

Under the watchful eye of the Queen Mother, girls who have had their first period are taken to an isolated place. During two to three weeks, the girl is initiated into the secrets of sexuality. Furthermore, she is told everything she needs to know about contraception and intercourse with men, and how she will be able to lead a good marriage and thus maintain her own dignity and the dignity of the community (Boakye 2009).

The care and preparation extended to young women in Akan society is entirely lacking in modern Western societies.

One reason for that is that archetypes of women, especially in modern cultures, have a foundation in a male ideal that is based on what men perceive they want, and don't want, from women. Confusing the issue even further is the fact that many archetypes in the modern world are manufactured by corporations. And regardless of what their public relation departments want you to believe, the primary interest of these billion dollar companies is twofold: to support the values of patriarchy and to make money.

The truth is that rarely do traditional or modern female archetypes offer young women role models that value self-worth or true liberation. Nor do they provide young women with a viable roadmap that will help them find satisfaction and fulfillment in their intimate relationships.

But what if a contemporary woman didn't have to struggle with self-limiting cultural archetypes? We believe that such a woman would be able to immerse herself in energy with universal qualities. That energy would have such a profound effect on her soul and spirit that she would be nourished and satisfied in a myriad of ways. Such a woman would do things that were appropriate for her regardless of the risks. She would view her body as a sacred temple worthy of honor and love. She would nourish it with wholesome foods and her physical activities would be a reflection of her self-love.

In the following pages, we will look at some life-affirming archetypes that could help women, especially those in puberty, to express their power, creativity, and radiance freely. After that, you will learn how to release self-limiting archetypes and replace them with life-affirming female archetypes that honor women and the universal qualities of the feminine.

## Archetypes for the Radiant Woman

The first archetype we will look at is Lilith.

According to Hebrew tradition, Lilith was Adam's first wife. She was not created from Adam's rib like Eve, his second wife, but was formed from the same clay that he was formed of, which at least in Lilith's mind made her Adam's equal.

> Lilith is this, Adam's first wife.
> Be aware of her beautiful hair,
> of this jewelry in which she shines.
> If she reaches the young man with it,
> she will not let go of him so easily.
>
> —J. W. V. GOETHE (1798)

Lilith was mentioned only once in the Old Testament (Joshua 34, 14). Other than that, she was completely banned from it. However, she was not banned from Hebrew tradition. From the Alphabet of Ben Sira, which entered Europe from the East in the sixth century AD, we learn that "as soon as she had been created, Lilith started an argument and said: 'Why should I lie beneath you? I am worthy as much as you are and we have both been created from the earth.'" (Humm 1995)

By refusing to submit to male authority, Lilith's relationship with Adam became so acrimonious that she decided to leave paradise.

Even though the Alphabet of Ben Sira pictured her as a highly sexual woman whose innate female power and radiance had an almost hypnotic effect on men, that view eventually changed. In medieval Hebrew society, it was argued by scholars that her erotic appeal was caused by the dark forces and demons that dominated her.

Of course, there is more than one version of the story. But the authors of the Talmud made it abundantly clear that Lilith had to go and that Adam needed a more submissive wife. So, they concocted the idea that Jehovah had mercy on Adam and created a second wife for him, Eve. No such mercy was extended to Lilith. Since that time, Lilith has been depicted in both Hebrew and Christian scripture as a winged demon, beautiful but cruel, and of course exceedingly toxic to any man who came in contact with her (Howe Gaines 2012).

## The Other Side of Lilith

To those women who yearn to overcome self-limiting archetypes, the insubordinate and freedom loving ancestral woman, who combines fertility and death, shadows and light, offers a model. She brings to the attention of women the dangers of weakness and conformity. She is a woman who isn't afraid to assert herself, who never surrenders, and who experiences and embraces her own sexuality.

Could it be that the archetype of Lilith provides women with a new identity based on freedom, power, and radiance? If so, perhaps it's Lilith who can guide you into the deepest corners of your unconscious in order to show you your ancestral femininity and strength. And if you are ready to embrace those qualities by seeing Lilith as a positive role model for women, you can reunite with them. Because you deserve what Lilith wanted to achieve, which was neither to stand above nor beneath men, but simply to be their equal.

## Shakti

Shakti provides another life-affirming archetype for the modern woman. In Indian society, Shakti's attributes are almost exclusively positive. That is because Indian society, which has been deeply influenced by the teachings of yoga and tantra, recognizes that a person's relationship to feminine energy has a deep and abiding influence on their well-being and the health of their relationships.

Shakti's origins can be traced back several thousand years. As an archetype of women and all that is creative in the universe, she has influenced Hinduism, Buddhism, and even some of the cults in ancient Greece and Rome, including the cult of Dionysus.

According to yoga and tantra, Shakti serves as a model for womanhood because she represents the primordial cosmic force that creates and sustains the universe. Among Hindus, Shakti is sometimes referred to as the Great Divine Mother.

On the earth plane, Shakti manifests her power most directly through women. Swamini Mayatitananda notes that "At the beginning of Creation...(Shakti)...took form and set in motion the wheel of manifestation. She bestowed her healing spirit and regenerative energy into the womb of every female of every species on earth."

In Hindu mythology, Shakti has taken on many forms that affirm the power, creativity, and radiance of women, including Parvati, the good wife, Durga, the nourishing mother, and Kali, the warrior supreme.

## Five Life-Affirming Archetypes

Although Lilith and Shakti offer archetypes that affirm the strength, creativity, and power of women, we've included five more life-affirming archetypes in this chapter. You can adopt any of them in the next series of exercises to replace the archetypes that have prevented you from expressing your power, creativity, and radiance freely.

### The Innocent Girl

This archetype can be adopted by any woman who has been traumatized or abused as a child. The most important qualities of the innocent girl are innocence and trust. To use this archetype in the next series of exercises, you must visualize yourself as a woman who has retained her innocence. You can represent this in your visualization by your posture, your expression, what you wear, and the symbolic items that you carry with you.

To be innocent doesn't mean to be naive or childish. Innocence is the purity of soul that a joyful, balanced woman retains throughout her life. It's lost when a woman's energy field has been contaminated by self-limiting archetypes and by projections from selfish and abusive people.

By trust, we mean more than the trust in a benevolent universe. In this context, trust includes the self-trust and confidence that can only emerge in a woman when she knows herself and takes the risk to be herself.

### The Warrior

This archetype can be adopted by any woman ready to take back her feminine power and to freely assert it once more in the world. The warrior is a woman who respects herself because she respects her intuition and what she senses about the world around her. The warrior has developed courage and perseverance. She has character because she has chosen to be herself regardless of the cost. As a result, she can't be manipulated by the core values of patriarchy, which equate femininity with weakness and dependence. The woman who becomes a warrior is the master of her own mind and the equal of any man.

To use the archetype of the warrior in the next series of exercises, visualize yourself with a firm gaze and in a pose that manifests power and self-confidence. The clothes you wear and the symbolic items you carry with you should symbolize your strengths and unique abilities.

### The Nourishing Woman

This archetype can be adopted by any woman who needs to overcome self-importance, narcissism, or the need for male attention. All these qualities emerge from patterns of self-doubt and insecurity that indicate a lack of self-esteem. The nourishing woman is someone who has more prana than necessary to sustain herself and those dependent on her.

To use this archetype in the next series of exercises, you should visualize yourself as a woman who is self-confident and looks inward while she radiates her excess feminine energy through her eyes and hands.

The nourishing woman doesn't require a man's validation to feel whole. She has a generous nature and radiates her nourishing power to both "saint and sinner alike." The nourishing woman has overcome the narcissism and egotism that comes from the inability to love herself and other people. Such a woman gives without expecting anything in return.

## The Adventurous Woman

This archetype can be adopted by any woman who feels trapped in a conventional life that is stifling her. If you feel like you're drowning in the needs of others and that you must sacrifice your own well-being for family or friends, the adventurous woman offers you a way to achieve the inner freedom that you seek. The adventurous woman doesn't run away from life; she embraces it by creating an inner life that is rich in adventure and experience.

If you're a woman who seeks her own path, the adventurous woman offers you the inner strength and conviction that will allow you to make your own decisions and create an ethic that puts the universal qualities of the feminine first. The adventurous woman has the courage to be herself. She risks the censor of others to follow her own path and to live with integrity.

The adventurous woman has discipline and perseverance. She trusts her senses and embraces all experiences, both good and bad. Such a woman learns from her mistakes and becomes stronger as a result. Although she may wander alone at times, she is never lonely because she has found herself.

To use this archetype in the next series of exercises, you should visualize yourself in a pose that manifests your courage and inner strength, as well as the inner freedom you experience.

## The Wise Woman

This archetype can be adopted by any woman who consistently makes bad decisions. The problems most women face as adults arise when they make decisions that interfere with their relationship to the universal feminine and to themselves. Such decisions are motivated by patterns that arise from concentrations of karmic baggage and subtle energetic attachments. That is why the universe doesn't support these decisions, and why they don't enhance the flow of prana through a woman's energy field.

Facts don't lie: When a woman's core values don't support her relationship to herself and to the universal feminine, then the decisions she makes will inevitably lead to pain and suffering. Decisions to love a wounded or abusive man, to sacrifice yourself for others, or to embrace a sexual persona that demeans a woman's dignity are examples of bad decisions. Wise women never make such decisions. Instead, they remain mindful and consistently make decisions based on values that enhance a woman's power, creativity, and radiance.

To use this archetype, visualize yourself as a self-confident woman who trusts her own feminine power and intuition. She has given up guilt and shame because she has learned from her mistakes. As a result, she feels prana flowing through her. And she never makes a decision that interrupts her relationship with this life-affirming energy. It's the wise woman of any age who can heal the world.

## Let's Get Practical

In the series of three exercises that follows, you will release a self-limiting archetype. Then you will use one of the life-affirming archetypes we've presented, or one of your own, to replace the archetype that you released.

Common cultural archetypes of girls and young women that are self-limiting include mommy's girl, daddy's girl, the princess, the outsider, the loser, the conformist, the rebel, the egotist, the slut, and the popular girl.

Although the popular girl appears to be a positive archetype, it's self-limiting because it puts a girl into an ill-fitting box. It also makes demands on a girl, which limit her choices and her ability to express herself fully.

Common cultural archetypes of women that are self-limiting include the Barbie doll, the trophy wife, the damaged woman, the man-eater, the dependent woman, and the nag. Once you've chosen a self-limiting archetype that we've provided, or one of your own, select one of the life-affirming archetypes that we've provided, or one of your own, to replace it.

In the first exercise, you will use the visual screen to release the self-limiting archetype you have in mind. In the second exercise, you will replace it with the life-affirming archetype of your choice. Then you will perform the Self-Esteem Mudra. The Self-Esteem Mudra will enhance your self-esteem, once you've replaced a self-limiting archetype with one that enhances your life-affirming identity.

---

## Exercise: Releasing a Self-Limiting Archetype

To begin the exercise, find a comfortable position with your back straight. Then breathe deeply through your nose for two to three minutes. Use the Standard Method to relax your muscles and to center yourself in your authentic mind. Then choose a self-limiting archetype to release and a life-affirming archetype to replace it. Keep both archetypes in mind.

Then create a visual screen in front of you by asserting, *"It's my intent to create a visual screen eight feet (two-and-a-half meters) in front of me."* Once the visual screen has materialized, assert, *"It's my intent to visualize myself personifying the self-limiting archetype I've chosen to release on the visual screen."* Immediately, you will see an image of the woman you don't want to be. Take a few moments to study the archetype. Observe how it makes you look. Empathize with it so that you can feel how the archetype has restricted your access to energy with universal qualities. When you're satisfied with what you've experienced, mentally draw a circle around the archetype and a red line through the circle. Then assert, *"It's my intent to release the archetype on the screen, and all the energy and consciousness in my energy field and physical body that support it."* Immediately, the archetype will disappear. Once it's gone, release the image of yourself and the screen by asserting, *"It's my intent to release the image of myself and the screen in front of me."* Then take ten minutes to enjoy the effects.

After ten minutes, count from one to five. Then open your eyes and bring yourself out of the exercise. You only have to release the self-limiting archetype once. In the next exercise, you will replace it with the life-affirming archetype of your choice.

---

## Exercise: Integration of a
## Life-Affirming Archetype

In this exercise, you will replace the self-limiting archetype you just released with a life-affirming archetype. To begin the exercise, find a comfortable position with your back straight. Then breathe deeply through your nose for two to three minutes. Use the Standard Method to relax your muscles and to center yourself in your authentic mind. Then bring to mind the life-affirming archetype that you've chosen to replace the self-limiting archetype you released in the last exercise.

To continue, assert, *"It's my intent to create a visual screen eight feet (two-and-a-half meters) in front of me."* As soon as the screen appears, assert, *"It's my intent to visualize myself on the screen personifying the life-affirming archetype I have in mind."* As soon as the image appears, observe her, how she carries herself, what radiates through her eyes. Take time to observe what she wears and if she has something to say or teach you. Once you're satisfied with what you've learned, assert, *"It's my intent to replace the archetype I released previously with the life-affirming archetype on the visual screen."* Don't do anything after that; just relax and for the next ten minutes, let the life-affirming archetype and her universal qualities take root in your energy field and body. After ten minutes, count from one to five and bring yourself out of the exercise. You can repeat the exercise until you feel satisfied that the changes you desire have taken root in your identity.

## Exercise: The Self-Esteem Mudra

After you've substituted a life-affirming archetype for a self-limiting archetype, you're ready to perform the Self-Esteem Mudra. The Self-Esteem Mudra will help you integrate the new archetype by enhancing your self-confidence and self-esteem.

To perform the mudra, sit in a comfortable position with your back straight. Use the Standard Method to relax your muscles and to center yourself in your authentic mind. Then form a cup with your hands. Next, place the sides of your thumbs together. Continue by placing your left index finger, from the tip to the first joint, over the tip of the right index finger as far as the first joint. Do the same with your middle fingers. Then put the tips of your ring fingers and the tips of your pinky fingers together. Press your tongue up against the roof of your mouth and slide it back until the roof becomes soft. Then put the soles of your feet together. Hold the mudra for ten minutes while you breathe in and out from your solar plexus. After ten minutes, release the mudra and open your eyes. Repeat as needed.

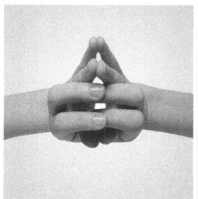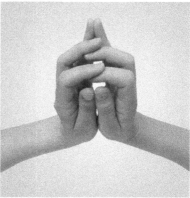

*Figure 10: The Self-Esteem Mudra*

## Summary

In this chapter, you learned how contaminated aspects of mind and man-made archetypes can disrupt the development of a life-affirming identity. Then you learned skills to release foreign aspects of mind and to heal your personal aspects of mind that were contaminated. In addition, you learned how to release self-limiting archetypes and replace them with life-affirming archetypes.

In the next chapter, you will learn why evolution favored the development of two human minds—a female mind and a male mind. And you will learn simple skills that will enable you to enhance the aspects of your authentic mind and energy field that make you uniquely feminine.

## SIX
# The Unique Female Mind

Although women and men have many things in common, it's only by recognizing the differences and the unique capabilities of the female mind that you can get an accurate picture of what you can achieve now that you've liberated yourself from restrictive beliefs and self-limiting archetypes.

The mind of all human beings is composed of three essential elements. On the physical level, it includes the brain and nervous system as well as the chemicals in the body, including hormones, that influence its structure and activities.

On the non-physical level, the mind includes the subtle energy field, its organs and vehicles, and the prana that nourishes them. The combination of physical and non-physical elements creates the third part of the human mind—the network. All three parts have their own unique capabilities and needs.

The network includes the connections the mind has to its individual parts and to things beyond itself. This includes consciousness and energy, as well as attachments to other people, non-physical beings, and their projections.

The organs of perception (sight, sensation, hearing, etc.) are also part of the human mind. They can be directed inward into the mind itself, or outward into the external environment. When they are directed outward, they can make contact with other networks and interact with them.

## A World with Two Minds

Scientists now recognize that nature favored the evolution of two minds, and that the female mind is superior to the male mind in performing complex tasks and reading emotional cues. The differences don't end there. There are significant differences in polarity, on the energetic level, that allow women to connect to the earth and its innate power in ways that most men can't. And there are the obvious hormonal differences that make women more nurturing, intuitive, empathetic, and giving.

Because of its unique qualities, particularly its ability to recognize emotional cues and its greater sensitivity to interactions of subtle energy, a woman's mind can also develop skills based on intuitive insight and the lessons learned from experience, in both the physical and non-physical universe. It can then solve problems concerning physical survival. And it can diagnose and heal psychic and spiritual problems using energy with universal qualities and the skill it has developed.

Another important aspect of a woman's mind barely recognized by modern societies is this: virtually every person alive today has incarnated on earth more than once. This means that most women have a personal history and karmic heritage that can span generations. A woman's unique personal history plays a significant role in how her mind functions, what she values, what talents she brings into this life, and how she expresses herself. In the body of this chapter, we will look at how a woman can enhance her unique functions of mind to increase her power, creativity, and radiance.

## Seeking Abundance

Because the polarity of a woman's mind differs in significant ways from a man's mind, a woman's spiritual relationship to the earth and the non-physical universe is different.

On the spiritual level, a man's mind is hard-wired to transcend the limitations of earthly existence in order to achieve peace and harmony.

In contrast, a woman's mind seeks to participate fully with the earth and integrate itself with the abundance of energy and life that emerges from it.

Abundance is only indirectly related to the acquisition of material things. In spiritual terms, abundance is more closely related to acquiring the essentials necessary to meet one's needs on the levels of spirit, soul, and body.

This holistic approach to life is natural for women. Indeed, without fulfilling her need for abundance, a woman's life will feel empty. And she will feel that she is not anchored properly to the earth and the energy that emerges from it. There is a good reason for this: a woman's physical-material chakras are masculine in relationship to the earth. This means that a woman actively reaches out to the earth with her subtle energy field and her functions of mind to connect to it.

In contrast, a man's physical-material chakras are feminine in relationship to the earth. This means men are receptive to the earth. And instead of actively reaching out to it, they merely accept the life force and energy freely offered to them.

Although women have a more complex relationship to the earth and have the desire to participate in its essential, life-giving qualities, modern societies don't enthusiastically support an active relationship between people and the life-giving earth.

In spite of this, you can reach out to the earth with your mind, as if it's a living thing, in order to receive the abundance from it that is your birthright. In order to achieve that, you will learn to perform the Meditation for Abundance.

---

### Exercise: Meditation for Abundance

In the Meditation for Abundance, you will strengthen your relationship to the earth by activating your physical-material chakras. Then you will center yourself in your upper and lower physical-material chakra fields. Once you are centered, you will enhance the masculine polarity of these chakra fields by centering yourself in the first polar field, which is assertive and therefore masculine. This will enable you to reach out to the earth and participate actively in the abundance of life and energy it has to offer you.

*Exercise*

To begin the meditation, find a comfortable position with your back straight. Breathe deeply through your nose for two to three minutes. Then count backward from five to one and from ten to one. Use the Standard Method to relax your muscles and to center yourself in your authentic mind. Then assert, *"It's my intent to activate my upper physical-material chakra."* Next, assert, *"It's my intent to activate my lower physical-material chakra."* Take a few moments to enjoy the shift. Then assert, *"It's my intent to center myself in my upper physical-material chakra field."* Continue by asserting, *"It's my intent to center myself in my lower physical-material chakra field."* Take a few moments to enjoy the enhanced flow of prana. Then assert, *"In my upper and lower physical-material chakras, it's my intent to center myself in my first polar field."*

Because your first polar field is masculine, by centering yourself in it you will radiate more intent, will, and desire through your physical-material chakras. That in turn will strengthen your connection to the earth.

Enjoy the enhanced connection you have to the earth and to the subtle energy emerging from it for fifteen minutes. Then count from one to five and bring yourself out of the meditation. Repeat as needed.

## The Female Brain

The physical part of the human mind includes the nervous system and brain as well as the chemicals in the body that support them. The brain controls many of the functions of the physical body and interacts with the other two elements of the human mind on a continuous basis. But not all brains are the same. The communication center is bigger in the female brain than in the male brain. So is the emotional memory center. The female brain develops a greater ability to read subtle, verbal and non-verbal cues in people than does the male brain.

Because of these differences, a woman's primary values are communication, connection, emotional sensitivity, and responsiveness. It's the differences in the female brain that explain why women prize these qualities above all others and why they are so often baffled by a person with a brain that doesn't grasp the importance of these qualities, namely a person with a male brain (Wolf 2005).

Although scientific discoveries have offered us insights into the role played by the brain and nervous system and the part that hormones play, until recently it was rare for science or any discipline, like psychology, biology, or philosophy, to take into consideration the obvious fact that a woman's brain differs from a man's brain.

Therefore with this patriarchal prejudice in mind, it's not surprising that there has been very little research into how changes in technology or societal norms disrupt the functions of a woman's brain and how these disruptions affect a woman's relationship to her family, to herself, and to the ecology of life that exists in the physical and non-physical universe.

## The Problem of Multi-Tasking

In the case of multi-tasking, this is particularly unfortunate. That's because the combination of activities in multi-tasking can interfere with the functions of a woman's brain and subtle energy field.

Researchers have described multi-tasking as a form of violence against the mind. That's because multi-tasking rewires the brain, so that in a short time a normal brain begins to resemble the brain of a person with an addictive personality (Hänsel 2012). This can be devastating for a woman and her relationships since the brain affects the network. And the network's primary activity is to perceive and communicate with people in a holistic way.

Holistic means that body language, the spoken word and the radiation of prana are perceived and interpreted by the brain and used by the subtle energy field, and the network, to create a complete experience.

Texting, chatting, computer games, and multi-tasking disrupt the normal chemistry of the brain and can cause so much stress for the subtle energy field that the network breaks down, along with normal perception and communication.

Multi-tasking not only disrupts normal brain chemistry and the human energy field, it disrupts the ability of the brain and subtle energy field to integrate their activities. This in turn can disrupt a woman's ability to prioritize, thus making it difficult for a woman to recognize what is important and what is not.

Given enough time, multi-tasking will disrupt the functions of the human energy system by blocking the flow of prana through the chakras and the minor energy centers in the hands and feet. This will prevent a woman from connecting with the earth and sharing in its abundance. And it will disrupt a woman's empathy and her ability to achieve and sustain intimacy.

Because multi-tasking can create so many problems for women, we've included the Core Field Meditation in this chapter. The Core Field Meditation will help you overcome the most disruptive aspects of multi-tasking so that you can continue to empathize with people and to share energy with universal qualities with them.

## The Core Field

The core field is one of several resource fields that interpenetrate your subtle energy field. There is very little literature, ancient or modern, concerning resource fields and their importance. However, in our work we've learned that while your sense of personal identity emerges from your energy bodies, sheaths, and subtle energy system, it's your resource fields that provide your subtle energy field and subtle energy system with the consciousness and energy they need to coordinate their activities and function healthfully.

In the Core Field Meditation, you will experience your functions of mind—intent, will, desire, resistance, surrender, acceptance, knowing, choice, commitment, rejection, faith, enjoyment, destruction, creativity, empathy, and love—as part of a large field of consciousness and energy that fills and surrounds your energy field. Once you're relaxed, you will center yourself in the core field. Then you will turn your organs of perception inward on the level of the core field. This will allow you to sense the core field clearly. In the next step, you will choose a function of mind that you need to enhance. Then you will use your intent to fill that section of the core field with prana.

---

## Exercise: Core Field Meditation

To begin the Core Field Meditation, find a comfortable position with your back straight. Then choose a function of mind you wish to enhance. We will use enjoyment as an example. After you've made your choice, close your eyes and breathe deeply through your nose for two to three minutes. Then count backward from five to one and from ten to one. Use the Standard Method to relax your muscles and to center yourself in your authentic mind. Then assert, *"It's my intent to center myself in my core field."* Continue by asserting, *"It's my intent to turn my organs of perception inward on the level of my core field."* Take a few moments to enjoy the shift. Then assert, *"It's my intent to fill my core field with prana in the section associated with enjoyment."* Take fifteen minutes to experience the shift in your core field. Then bring yourself out of the meditation by counting from one to five. When you reach the number five, open your eyes. You will feel wide-awake, perfectly relaxed, and better than you did before. Repeat as needed.

## Hunters and Gatherers

Hunters (men) and gatherers (women) needed different mental capabilities to enhance survival. This explains why some men surpass women in some cognitive abilities, e.g., spatial sense, mathematical conclusions, orientation, and target-oriented motor abilities—all useful abilities if you're a hunter. Women, on the other hand, often have better verbal skills and perceive things more quickly. In many cases, they can remember certain details of a path more easily and they can often accomplish precision tasks much faster—all useful if you gather food and are responsible for maintaining the family and cultural continuity.

Sexual hormones are responsible for many of these differences as well as the ability many women have to read subtle facial and emotional expressions and cues.

Recent research by Dr. Christiane Northrup, an American gynecologist and a leading authority in the field of women's health and wellness, has found something remarkable about the female mind. Because of the influence of hormones, the corpus callosum in women is larger and thicker than in men. The corpus callosum is the part of the brain that connects the right and left hemispheres.

On a functional level, this means that women know or gain knowledge by experiencing something in both their centers of cognition and in their body at the same time. What this means, on a practical level, is that a woman's body and mind are on the same page at the same time and that the average woman has a more developed body intelligence than the average man (Walker 2007).

Although the influence of sexual hormones can have many positive effects, a disruption in the balance of a woman's sex hormones can cause the brain to fall into a depressive state for several months and the network to withdraw from many interactions on the energetic level. This can be exacerbated by early childhood programming, trauma, and projections from other people. Because depression in Western society has reached epidemic proportions, we've included an Anti-Depression Meditation in this chapter.

### Exercise: Anti-Depression Meditation

The Anti-Depression Meditation should be performed once a day, preferably in the morning, until the symptoms of depression have disappeared.

To begin the Anti-Depression Meditation, find a comfortable position with your back straight. Then close your eyes and breathe deeply through your nose for two to three minutes. Count backward from five to one and from ten to one. Then use the Standard Method to relax your muscles and to center yourself in your authentic mind.

Once you're relaxed, focus your mental attention on the right side of your brain for two to three minutes. Next, focus your mental attention on the left side of your brain for two to three minutes. Try to detect differences between the two hemispheres. Check the temperature. Does one side feel warmer than the other? Is there more pressure on one side than the other? Is one side of your brain numb while the other side is not? Are there localized feelings of discomfort on one side of your brain and not the other? Take as long as you need to detect the differences. Then use your right thumb to firmly press the acupuncture point at the top of your head for ten seconds After ten seconds, release the pressure and wait for ten seconds. Repeat three times.

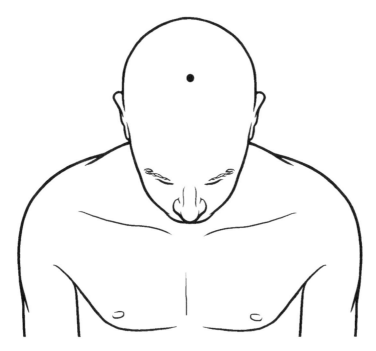

*Figure 11: The Acupuncture Point at the Top of the Head*

By stimulating the acupuncture point, you will enhance the flow of prana through your brain and through your sixth and seventh chakras. To enhance the flow of prana even further, you can assert, *"It is my intent to enhance the flow of prana through my brain so that balance and harmony are restored."* Take fifteen minutes to enjoy the process. Then count from one to five. When you reach the number five, open your eyes and bring yourself out of the meditation. Repeat as needed.

## Karmic Baggage and the Mind

A woman's karmic heritage in the form of karmic baggage from this life and past lives can have a negative impact on a woman's mind by creating attachments that disrupt the functions of her subtle energy system (chakras, auras, meridians, and minor energy centers).

As you learned in chapter 4, karmic baggage is the dense, self-limiting energy with individual qualities that women (and men) carry in their subtle energy field from one lifetime to another.

Attachments, created by karmic baggage, can influence a woman's subtle energy field, and therefore her mind, in three ways: they can restrict a woman's access to prana, they can create restrictive patterns (personality issues) that are not an essential part of a woman's mind, and they can keep a woman attached to people and relationship issues that remain unresolved from childhood and/or past lives.

Although the projection of aspects of mind can cause attachments in most cases, attachments to other people take the form of cords. Cords closely resemble long, thin tubes that have a consistent diameter along their entire length. When a person has become attached to karmic baggage in their energy field and then projects it in the form of a cord, it can get stuck in their target's energy field. When that happens, an attachment will be created that will connect the perpetrator to his or her target as long as the perpetrator holds on to the false impression that he or she needs or wants something from the target.

Another thing about cords is that they don't disappear when the perpetrator and/or target dies. This means that you can remain attached to someone from a past life, in most cases a past life lover, for lifetimes if she or he projected a cord into your energy field. And that connection can interfere with your ability to share the universal qualities of the feminine with the people you love in this life.

It's important to recognize that, like you, your past life lovers are inter-dimensional beings. When they die, they don't just disappear along with their karmic baggage and the cords they've projected. After a pause, they are reincarnated into a new body. That means you can remain attached to a past life lover for lifetimes, and that attachment can create a yearning in you for one or more of their most compelling qualities.

Of course, if your lover is dead, you won't find him or her. Even if he or she is incarnated, your past life lover is probably the wrong age, or living on the other side of the world. It's also possible that you may not want the lover anymore even if you found him or her, because the two of you have evolved in different directions. In any case, remaining attached to a past life lover and/or one of their qualities will disrupt the functions of your energy field, and prevent you from integrating the three elements of your mind to create a full experience.

Fortunately, even if you don't remember your past life lover, you can overcome your attachment by severing the cord that continues to connect you together.

You may wonder how you can overcome an attachment to someone who's dead and who you don't remember. However, it's possible. In fact, you don't have to know his or her name or what your past life lover looked like. You don't even have to know exactly what kind of relationship you had. All you have to do is to isolate the quality you've been yearning for, or the quality that is disrupting your ability to share prana with someone you love. If you do that, you'll isolate the cord your past life lover projected into your field. When you've isolated the cord, you can sever the energetic link that attaches you by using the appropriate functions of mind.

## Lena's Story

Lena's story illustrates how an attachment to a past life lover, created by a cord, can interfere with a woman's life and relationships.

In her first session with us, Lena, a thirty-one-year-old woman from Hamburg, explained that she'd recently met a man who was exactly her type. In fact, the attraction was so intense that she decided to sleep with him on the first date.

The date began with dinner at one of Hamburg's finest restaurants. After dinner, Lena and her friend returned to her apartment where they shared some wine and began to pet one another. But even though she was living her romantic dream, Lena still couldn't relax. Her muscles remained tense. And she knew that her body language was putting out conflicting signals. She managed to consummate the relationship that night, even though penetration caused her pain and she continued to behave awkwardly.

After relating the story, Lena told us that she'd never been able to let go and enjoy sex with a man. When we examined her energy field at the end of the session, we discovered that a cord attached Lena to a past life lover. The cord was located at one of the worst places possible, by her second chakra.

We released the cord in her next session, and almost immediately Lena felt a renewed sense of receptivity and well-being. After the session, we explained that the second chakra blockage had prevented her subtle energy system from distributing prana freely, and that without enough prana, she wouldn't have been able to have a satisfying sexual experience with a man.

---

## Exercise: Severing a Past Life Connection

To release a cord that connects you to a past life lover, you will begin by choosing a feeling you yearn for or a blockage that consistently interferes with your ability to share the universal qualities of the feminine with another person. After you've chosen a feeling or blockage, find a comfortable position with your back straight. Then close your eyes and breathe deeply through your nose for two to three minutes. Count backward from five to one and from ten to one. Then use the Standard Method to relax your muscles and to center yourself in your authentic mind. Once you are relaxed, assert, *"It's my intent to create a visual screen eight feet (two-and-a-half meters) in front of me."* As soon as the screen appears, perform the Orgasmic Bliss Mudra and hold it. Then assert, *"It's my intent to become aware of the cord that is responsible for the (feeling or blockage here) I've chosen to release."* Take a moment to observe the cord. It will be long and thin and will extend from your energy field all the way into the perpetrator's energy field. After you've examined the cord, assert, *"It's my intent to create a prana box around the cord I have in mind."* Then assert, *"It's my intent to fill the prana box with bliss and to release the cord and its source and extensions."* As soon as the cord has been released, you will feel a shift in your energy field. Pressure will diminish. Prana will flow more freely. And you will be able to remain centered in your authentic mind more easily. Like Lena, you may also experience a renewed sense of well-being and softer feelings emerging from your energy field.

Once you've released the cord, release the prana box and the visual screen. Release the mudra next. Then take ten minutes to enjoy the effects. After ten minutes, count from one to five and open your eyes. You will feel wide-awake, perfectly relaxed, and better than you did before.

You can use the same technique to release cords that attach you to people in this life as well as from past lives. Repeat as needed.

## Summary

In this chapter, you learned that a woman's mind is composed of three parts and that each part has unique capabilities and needs. You also learned exercises designed to overcome depression, enhance your connection to the earth, protect you from the most disruptive effects of multi-tasking, and to release attachments to past life lovers.

In the next chapter, you will learn how passive-aggressive patterns can prevent you from manifesting your power in healthy ways. Then you will learn to enhance your power by embracing the middle way, and by releasing the passive-aggressive patterns that continue to disrupt your life and relationships.

# SEVEN
## *Enhancing Female Power*

In earlier generations, the acculturation process and unequal expectations, opportunities, rewards, and punishments instilled in both women and men the belief that it was natural for men to have more power than women. This imbalance was one of the most common features of many societies and their institutions, until the twenty-first century.

But this imbalance could not be enforced solely through violence, discriminatory laws, and a repressive social contract. These societies, many of which oppressed men as well as women, also needed to have people accept their core values. To do that, they assigned a list of human characteristics according to gender (gender roles), which both women and men were expected to accept without question and integrate into their lives.

Many of these societies demanded that women should be nurturing, gentle, receptive, patient, chaste, attractive, in touch with their feelings, etc. These attributes are natural to women, and to men, too. But until recently, societies in Europe, the Middle East, and North America demanded that women accept them as core values while many men, especially those in authority, were free to reject them in order to embrace another set of values which they were taught were the sole province of men. These included competitiveness, assertiveness, ambition, rationality, toughness, aggression, etc.

When someone didn't accept the attributes assigned to them, they often suffered ridicule, rejection, persecution, or worse, violence. All of this, including restrictive beliefs and early childhood programming, conspired to undermine a person's ability to express their power naturally. Since core values change slowly, this means that many people and institutions still adhere to values that make it difficult for women to embrace their feminine power and achieve their potential.

## The Middle Way

In this chapter, we will explain that there is an alternative to the gender attributes that are still assigned to women even in the twenty-first century. This alternative is the middle way: a balanced life that includes empathy and the power to express yourself and the universal qualities of the feminine freely.

By embracing the middle way, a woman will be able to perform as well as a man, or even better, in any job or productive activity, because she will have enough power and energy to support her progress and guarantee her success. It's by embracing the middle way that a woman will achieve her goals without the legacy of the past getting in the way.

However, before we begin our exploration of the middle way, it will be useful to remember that the power and freedom to express it that men take for granted was not always available to women. In fact, negative myths about women remind us how difficult it was for women to embrace their feminine power and to express themselves honestly in the past.

## Negative Myths about Empowerment

Ancient Greece, the birthplace of modern Western civilization, was unusually prolific when it came to negative myths about powerful women. Medusa, whose gaze could turn men to stone, the women of the Greek island of Lesbos, and the Amazons who made war against men, quickly come to mind. So does Circe, who seduced men and stripped them of their male power, and the Sirens whose song drove even the most powerful men mad.

Of course, the Greeks were not alone in their antipathy toward powerful women. The early Britons also saw strong women as a threat. Morgan, the sister of King Arthur, immediately comes to mind. Morgan was a powerful woman. But for men trapped in a medieval mindset, it was more convenient to cast her as a conniving, power-hungry witch than a powerful, radiant woman.

In a modern society, a radiant woman with power may not be compared to Medusa, who turned men to stone, or Morgan, who enchanted them and stripped them of their power, but she can be judged harshly when she tries to assert power. If a woman is powerful and manages to become successful in a man's world, she runs the risk of being labeled tough, conniving, angry, or worse, a ball-buster.

Although these unflattering myths and adjectives can still be used to undermine powerful women and discourage them from aspiring to positions of authority, none of these myths or adjectives describe real people. Rather they pander to men's irrational fear of liberated women and their innate power.

Nonetheless, these myths have had their effect. They undermine the natural aspirations of many young women. And they support passive-aggressive personality patterns that undermine women's trust in themselves and their feminine power.

## The Scold's Bridle

In the Middle Ages, a time when women had few ways to assert power in a healthy way, a woman found guilty of trying to influence her husband passive-aggressively by nagging could be forced to wear a scold's bridle.

The scold's bridle was a metal and leather device that fit over the mouth and was fixed in the back. It had a tongue depressor with spurs or sharp edges. When it went into the woman's mouth, it made talking painful. The device was meant to humiliate a woman convicted by a council of men for nagging. Sometimes, a scold's bridle had a chain attached to the front, so the victim could be led through the streets or tied to a post.

The scold's bridle was used throughout Europe and even in America until the seventeenth century. In some cases, all a husband had to do was accuse his wife of nagging and the mask was put on her. Women who disagreed with their husbands, or who were found guilty of cruel gossip or any other minor offense, could also be forced to wear a scold's bridle.

## Passive-Aggressive Games

Given that the core values that support rigid gender roles still manifest themselves in the media, education, and in the attitudes embraced by many families, it's no wonder that many people continue to embrace patterns of passive-aggressive behavior.

There are many passive-aggressive games that modern women still play. We've listed three of the most common. You will probably recognize at least one of them from your own experience or the experience of your friends and family members.

### Seduction

This can be a form of sexual play or a form of manipulation. Unfortunately, in many societies, women are taught that it's natural to use seduction to get what they want from men. Even today, in many societies, by using seduction to manipulate a man, a woman will block her access to the power that would normally emerge from her subtle energy field.

### Nagging

Women who are frustrated or who have learned as children to nag their parents will often continue to nag their partner or other men in their family to get what they want. Nagging is an extreme expression of powerlessness. And any woman who resorts to this pattern will suffer from a lack of self-esteem because she will be unable to express her authentic power freely.

### Guilt Trips

Some women who feel powerless will use a man's weakness or some manifestation of bad character to make him feel guilty. A guilt trip is dangerous because it disrupts intimacy and creates an environment that will inevitably destroy the trust and love necessary to keep partners together.

## Overcoming Passive-Aggressive Patterns

If you think you've mastered at least one passive-aggressive pattern and continue to use it in order to assert power and get what you want, you can perform the two exercises that follow. The first is called archetype bumping. And the second is called the Governor Meridian Meditation.

In archetype bumping, you will replace the passive-aggressive archetype you've integrated into your personality with a life-affirming archetype that enhances your power, creativity, and radiance. In the Governor Meridian Meditation, you will enhance your power by enhancing the flow of prana though your governor meridian.

---

## Exercise: Archetype Bumping

To begin archetype bumping, choose a passive-aggressive pattern that you've mastered, but would like to release. Then choose a life-affirming archetype to replace it (a list of life-affirming archetypes can be found in chapter 5). After you've chosen a pattern and an archetype to replace it, keep them both in mind. Next find a comfortable position with your back straight. Then close your eyes and breathe deeply through your nose for two to three minutes. Count backward from five to one and from ten to one. Then use the Standard Method to relax your muscles and to center yourself in your authentic mind. Continue by asserting, *"It's my intent to visualize a screen eight feet (two-and-a-half meters) in front of me."* As soon as the screen appears, assert, *"It's my intent to visualize myself on the screen acting out the passive-aggressive pattern I want to release and holding a sign in front of my chest that identifies the pattern clearly."* For example, if nagging is the passive-aggressive pattern you want to release, then the image should hold a sign that says "nagging woman."

Continue by drawing a black circle around the image of yourself on the screen. Then immediately delete it by drawing a red line through it. At the same time you're deleting the image, assert, *"It's my intent to release the passive-aggressive pattern I have in mind and all the qualities that support it."* Once you've released the passive-aggressive pattern, you will replace it with the life-affirming archetype you've chosen. To do that, assert, *"It's my intent to replace the passive-aggressive archetype I just released with the archetype of the (your archetype here)."* Empathize with the image for fifteen minutes and experience all the life-affirming qualities of the archetype taking root in your energy field and body. After fifteen minutes, release the image and the screen. Then count from one to five to bring yourself out of the meditation. Repeat as needed.

## The Governor Meridian

The Governor Meridian is the most important masculine meridian in the human energy system. It originates at the perineum, at the base of the spine, and extends upward along the spine to the seventh chakra at the crown of your head and beyond. The masculine parts of the seven traditional chakras are connected to it.

By performing the Governor Meridian Meditation, you will do two things that will empower you. You will increase the amount of assertive energy you have available by enhancing the flow of prana up your back. And you will enhance your self-confidence by balancing the flow of prana up the back of your body, which is masculine, with the flow of prana down the front of your body, which is feminine.

---

## Exercise: Governor Meridian Meditation

To begin the Governor Meridian Meditation, find a comfortable position with your back straight. Close your eyes and breathe deeply through your nose for two to three minutes. Then count backward from five to one and from ten to one. Use the Standard Method to relax your muscles and to center yourself in your authentic mind. Then assert, *"It's my intent to activate the back of my first chakra."* To activate the back of the chakra further, bring your mental attention to the chakra and breathe into it. Once the back of your first chakra begins to vibrate or to glow, slowly move your mental attention and breath upward from the back of your first chakra along the governor meridian until you reach the back of your second chakra. When you reach the back of your second chakra, assert, *"It's my intent to activate the back of my second chakra."* Enjoy the vibration and glow that emerges from the back of your second chakra for a few moments. Then continue in the same way, working upward along the governor meridian, until you've activated the back of all seven traditional chakras.

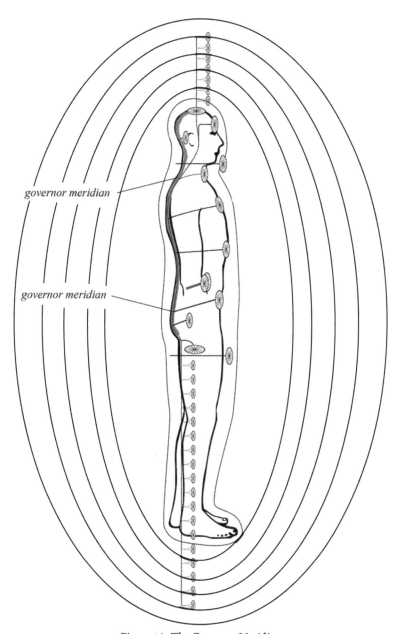

*Figure 12: The Governor Meridian*

Once you've activated the back of the seven traditional chakras, as-sert, *"It's my intent to center myself in my chakra fields on the level of my seven traditional chakras."* Take fifteen minutes to enjoy the experience. After fifteen minutes, count from one to five and bring yourself out of the meditation. Repeat as needed.

By activating the back of the seven traditional chakras and enhanc-ing the flow of prana through the governor meridian, you will enhance your personal power. That will enable you to express yourself as you really are, and not as other people want you to be.

Another way in which you can enhance your personal power and at the same time move forward and make progress in the world is to enhance the flow of prana through your minor energy centers in your hands and feet. You already learned to activate your minor energy cen-ters in chapter 3. In the two exercises that follow, you will take the next step by activating the minor energy centers in your hands and feet and by enhancing the flow of prana through the ruling meridians that sup-port them. To do that, we must first take a closer look at the system of meridians and how you can use it to empower yourself.

## Major Meridians

As you learned in chapter 3, meridians are streams of prana that have two important functions: They connect the chakras and minor energy cen-ters, scattered throughout your energy system, to one another. And they transmit prana to the parts of the human energy field where it's needed most. Although there are hundreds of important meridians, both ancient Chinese and Indian texts agree that there are ten ruling meridians: two of them are connected directly to the minor energy centers in the hands and two are connected directly to the minor energy centers in the feet. Yang meridians carry prana away from the center of the body while Yin merid-ians carry prana toward the center of your body.

### *The Yang Yu*

The two Yang Yu meridians are your masculine arm channels, located in both arms. They link your shoulders with the energy centers in your palms, after passing through the middle fingers.

*The Yin Yu*

The two Yin Yu are feminine arm channels, which link the centers in the palms with the chest. They travel along the insides of each arm. And along with the Yang Yu, they form the minor energy centers in the palms.

*The Yang Chiao*

The two Yang Chiao meridians rise from a central point in the soles of your feet and pass through the outer sides of your ankles and legs where they connect with additional meridians at the base of the penis-vagina.

*The Yin Chiao*

The two Yin Chiao meridians rise from a central point in the soles of the feet and pass through the inside of the ankles and legs where they connect with additional meridians at the base of the penis-vagina. They are called negative leg channels because they are Yin in relation to the Yang Chiao meridians. Along with the Yang Chiao meridians, they form minor energy centers in your feet.

It's these meridians, the Yang Yu—Yin Yu and the Yang Chiao—Yin Chiao, along with your energy centers in your hands and feet, which you will activate in the exercises that follow. By activating these organs, you will empower yourself to manifest your talents and strengths through your work and relationships. And you will empower yourself to move forward and make progress in the world.

---

## Exercise: Yin Yu and Yang Yu Meditations

The Yin Yu—Yang Yu Meditation is designed to enhance the flow of prana through the circuit formed by the meridians converging in your palms, first on the right side of your body and then on the left.

To begin the Yin Yu—Yang Yu Meditation, find a comfortable position with your back straight. Then use the Standard Method to relax your muscles and to center yourself in your authentic mind. Continue by asserting, *"It's my intent to activate my heart chakra."* Next, assert, *"It's my intent to center myself in my heart chakra field."* Once you're centered in your heart chakra field, assert, *"It's my intent to project my mental attention to the upper end of the Yang Yu meridian on the right side of my body."* If there are no obstructions, the moment your mental attention reaches the Yang Yu, the prana flowing through the meridian will carry it down the meridian to its terminus in the palm of the hand. As soon as your mental attention reaches the terminus, move it about an inch (two-and-a-half centimeters) diagonally down toward the base of your hand. This is the access point of the Yin Yu meridian (in your right palm). If there are no obstructions, the moment your mental attention finds the meridian, your attention will be carried up the inside of your arm (by the prana flowing through the meridian) to its terminus on the right side of your chest.

Once the circuit has been completed, release your mental attention and enjoy the enhanced flow of prana through the Yin Yu and Yang Yu meridians and through your energy center in your palm.

When you're ready to proceed to the second part of this exercise, assert, *"It's my intent to project my mental attention to the access point of the Yang Yu meridian on the left side of my body."* If there are no obstructions, the moment you locate the access point with your mental attention, it will be carried down to the meridian's terminus in the palm of the left hand. Continue by moving your mental attention one inch (two-and-a-half centimeters) diagonally down the palm, at a forty-five degree angle away from your thumb. There you'll find the access point of the Yin Yu meridian. Let the prana flowing through the meridian carry your mental attention to the terminus in the chest. Then release your mental attention.

Take fifteen minutes to enjoy the effects of the exercise. Then count from one to five. When you reach the number five open your eyes. You will feel wide-awake, perfectly relaxed, and better than you did before. If you practice this exercise everyday for as little as five days, you will experience a significant improvement in your motivation and your ability to manifest your feminine power in the world.

# Exercise: The Chao Yin—
## Chao Yang Meditation

In the Chao Yin—Chao Yang Meditation, you will enhance the flow of prana through the circuit formed by the meridians converging in the feet, first on the right side of your body space and then on the left. As the flow of prana through each circuit increases, your minor energy centers will become more active and you will be able to move forward and make more progress in the world.

To begin the exercise, find a comfortable position with your back straight. Then use the Standard Method to relax your muscles and to center yourself in your authentic mind. Continue by asserting, *"It's my intent to activate my heart chakra."* Next, assert, *"It's my intent to center myself in my heart chakra field."* Once you're centered in your heart chakra field, assert, *"It's my intent to project my mental attention to the upper end of the Chao Yang meridian on the right side of my body."* As soon as your mental attention has been projected to the access point of the Chao Yang, prana flowing through the meridian will carry it down to its terminus in the sole of your foot. Once your mental attention reaches the terminus, move your mental attention diagonally back and inside about an inch (two-and-a-half centimeters). This is the access point of the Chao Yin meridian (in the right sole). If there are no obstructions, the moment your mental attention finds the meridian, your attention will be carried up the inside of your ankle and thigh to a point one-and-a-half inches (four centimeters) below the base of the spine on the inside of your leg. Once the circuit has been completed, release your mental attention. Remain centered in your heart chakra field and enjoy the enhanced flow of prana in the sole center and the Chao Yang and Chao Yin meridians.

When you're ready to proceed, assert, *"It's my intent to project my mental attention to the access point of the Chao Yang meridian on the left side of my body."* If there are no obstructions, the moment your mental attention reaches the Chao Yang, the prana flowing through the meridian will carry it down to its terminus in the sole of your foot. Once your mental attention reaches the terminus, move your mental attention to the Chao Yin access point on the sole of the foot diagonally across and back about an inch (two-and-a-half centimeters). The moment your mental attention finds the meridian, it will be carried up the inside of your ankle and thigh to a point about one-and-a-half inches (four centimeters) below the base of your spine (by the prana flowing through the meridian). Once the circuit is complete, release your mental attention.

Take fifteen minutes to enjoy the effects of the exercise. Then count from one to five. When you reach the number five, open your eyes. You will feel wide-awake, perfectly relaxed, and better than you did before. If you practice this exercise everyday for as little as five days, you will experience a significant improvement in your motivation and your ability to make progress in the world.

## Summary

In the beginning of this chapter, you learned how passive-aggressive patterns can disrupt your power. And you learned to overcome passive-aggressive patterns by performing archetype bumping and the governor meridian meditation.

Later in the chapter, you learned to perform the Yin Yu—Yang Yu and the Chao Yin—Chao Yang Meditations. These two meditations, if practiced regularly, will enable you to manifest more of your power in the world—and make greater progress in your work and relationships.

In the following chapter, you will learn to enhance your creativity by enhancing your ability to conceive and manifest your creative ideas in the world.

# EIGHT
## *Enhancing Creativity*

Although everybody has the innate ability to be creative, few people can explain exactly what creativity is or how to fully manifest it in the physical world. What we do know intuitively is that a grandmother knitting a sweater for her grandchild is engaging in a creative act. So is a woman creating a new Internet-based business. Drafting a business proposal can be as creative as writing a symphony.

Creativity is only loosely related to talent. And although not everyone has talent in a particular field of endeavor, such as music or mathematics, everyone has vast resources of creativity lying dormant within them.

In the following pages, we will provide you with exercises to enhance your creativity so that it can blossom in any environment. But first you need to know that creativity is composed of two parts: conception and manifestation. Conception is supported by consciousness. It's consciousness that will enhance your receptivity to new concepts, interpretations, and ideas.

Manifestation, the ability to manifest your conception in the physical world, is the second part of the creative process. It requires you to recover your inner voice.

Although a woman's inner voice is the most important element of the creative process, nothing creative will take place unless a woman has access to the consciousness that she needs to support it. In order to help you access all the consciousness you need, we've included the Purusha Field Meditation. In this meditation, you will center yourself in the field of purusha, the primordial field of consciousness.

The purusha field is a resource field that emerged along with the field of prakriti, the primordial field of feminine energy, during the fourth tattva, the fourth step in the evolution of the universe. By practicing the Purusha Field Meditation, you will be accessing consciousness at its source. This will help you avoid much of the distortion that subsequently entered the diverse fields of consciousness during the later stages of evolution.

---

## Exercise: Purusha Field Meditation

To begin the Purusha Field Meditation, find a comfortable position with your back straight. Breathe deeply through your nose for two to three minutes. Then count backward from five to one and from ten to one. Use the Standard Method to relax your muscles and to center yourself in your authentic mind. Then assert, *"It's my intent to center myself in my purusha field."* Next, assert, *"It's my intent to fill my purusha field with prana."* Take a few moments to enjoy the shift. Then assert, *"It's my intent to turn my organs of perception inward on the level of my purusha field."*

Take fifteen minutes to enjoy the meditation. Then count from one to five. When you reach the number five, open your eyes. You will feel wide-awake, perfectly relaxed, and better than you did before.

By practicing the Purusha Field Meditation regularly, you will quickly recover the consciousness you need to support the creative process.

## Enhancing Intuition and Insight

Manifestation begins with the emergence of a woman's inner voice. Unfortunately, many women have become so bogged down and dependent on the opinions of other people—their parents, friends, bosses, etc.—that they rarely experience their inner voice. Other women, as part of early childhood programming, have learned to distrust their inner voice because they've been taught to give greater weight to the opinions and beliefs of people in positions of authority. The mass media also discourages women, especially young women entering puberty, from trusting their inner voice and from manifesting their creativity in the world.

Add to all that the lack of healthy female archetypes and the fact that many women have difficulty becoming fully autonomous, and it comes as no surprise that many women have difficulty feeling themselves and experiencing their inner voice.

## A Woman's Rite of Passage

In matriarchal societies, autonomy and the full emergence of a young woman's inner voice and creativity takes place at puberty and is celebrated in the rituals of a young woman's rite of passage. But in modern technological societies, where there is no clearly defined rite of passage into full womanhood, a young woman's inner voice can be disrupted in childhood by a mother or father whose psychological development remained incomplete and who is not fully autonomous. An overly protective parent, who has not achieved full autonomy, will smother his or her daughter with projections of distorted energy. And these projections can disrupt the daughter's access to her inner voice and innate creativity.

An overly possessive parent who has not achieved full autonomy will prevent his or her daughter from developing a strong life-affirming identity. Without a strong life-affirming identity, a young woman will lack the independence, self-esteem, and perseverance she needs to claim her inner voice as her own.

A parent who has not achieved full autonomy, who neglects his or her daughter and doesn't provide her with the love or nourishment she needs, will prevent her from developing the inner resources she needs to venture into the world alone. Fortunately, regardless of a woman's personal history, she can still reclaim her inner voice. That's because every woman has access through her energy field to the consciousness and energy she needs to overcome any obstacle that would restrict or inhibit her creativity and her ability to manifest it in the world.

# Julie's Story

The story of Julie illustrates how an overly possessive mother can disrupt a young woman's ability to access her inner voice. Julie was twenty-seven when she came to us for help. She'd been living in Freiburg, in Germany's Black Forest, since she'd graduated from the University of Heidelberg in 2008.

Julie grew up in a single parent home with a mother who was obsessed with cleanliness. Gudrun was controlling in other ways, too. And she was easily stressed when Julie was too loud or rambunctious.

As Julie grew up, she became more withdrawn and dependent on her mother's approval. She was loath to disobey her or even to express her own feelings and emotions. It wasn't long before fear began to dominate her life. Truth be told, she'd become an extension of her mother. As a result, she hadn't developed an independent identity or established healthy relationships with other children.

It was clear that her mother had never established an identity of her own, and that she'd poured her energy into her daughter in an effort to live vicariously through her. When Julie finished secondary school, on the advice of her mother, she became a lawyer, a profession that required very little human contact or creativity. However, unexpected problems began to emerge when she began dating a filmmaker from Berlin.

Through their intimate interactions, Peter recognized that Julie had become so dependent on her mother that she'd lost access to her inner voice. He inspired her to leave her mother behind and get help. That's when Julie came to us.

We immediately recognized that Julie had weak boundaries and that her chakra fields had been filled by her mother's subtle energetic projections. We also concluded that Julie's mother had disrupted her daughter's will, desire, and resistance, which meant that her mother had projected distorted energy from her own karmic baggage into Julie's core field.

Helping Julie establish an independent identity was our first priority. We taught her to heal her aspects of mind and to center herself in the appropriate resource fields. And within a few months, Julie could sense herself again. We continued by providing her with a series of tasks to regain her inner voice.

Julie has made great progress. And you can, too. If you've lost contact with your inner voice, you can regain it by performing the same series of tasks that helped Julie.

### The First Task

In order to reclaim your inner voice, your first task will be to let go of the inner drama you've absorbed from your mother or father. It's this drama and the karmic baggage that supports it which disrupts a woman's inner voice and creativity. That's because it internalizes values that devalue the universal qualities of the feminine and also creates an inner struggle that disrupts the formation of a strong and stable identity, which is necessary for a woman to express her creativity freely.

To accomplish your first task, you will perform the Infinite Freedom Meditation.

---

### Exercise: The Infinite Freedom Meditation

To begin the Infinite Freedom Meditation, find a comfortable position with your back straight. Close your eyes and breathe deeply through your nose for two to three minutes. Then count backward from five to one and from ten to one. Use the Standard Method to relax your muscles and to center yourself in your authentic mind. Then visualize a screen about eight feet (two-and-a-half meters) in front of you. Using your finger, draw a horizontal infinity symbol on the screen. Once you've drawn the infinity symbol, assert, *"It's my intent to visualize my mother within the left side of the infinity symbol."* Continue by asserting, *"It's my intent to visualize an image of myself within the right side of the infinity symbol."* Then assert, *"It's my intent to sever all the attachments to my mother that have disrupted my access to my inner voice."* Next, visualize a sword in your masculine hand, right hand if you're right-handed, left hand if you're left-handed. And with a quick and decisive stroke, cut the infinity symbol apart at its narrowest point. Then release the infinity symbol and the images of yourself and your mother. Release the screen next.

Then take about ten minutes to experience the shift. After ten minutes, count from one to five and open your eyes. When you open your eyes, you will feel wide-awake, perfectly relaxed, and you will recognize that control of your energy field is shifting back to you—where it belongs! Repeat as needed.

### The Second Task

For a woman to reclaim her inner voice, her second task will be to create more space in her energy field for her authentic emotions to be expressed.

The first chakra provides the prana that supports authentic emotions. Without this energy, emotions won't emerge freely. The second through sixth chakras and the auric fields that surround them regulate the expression of the four authentic human emotions: anger, fear, pain, and joy.

Although it may appear that all emotions are the same, the truth is that there are only four authentic emotions.

Emotions are authentic for three reasons: they're composed of energy with universal qualities, they emerge from your energy system via your chakras when your relationship to someone has been disrupted, and they can be resolved by screaming, yelling, crying, or by just letting the emotional energy rise upward to the organs of expression in your face.

In contrast to the four authentic emotions, there are a myriad of inauthentic emotions that can emerge from karmic baggage and external projections.

An emotion is inauthentic for two reasons: it emerges from fields of energy with individual qualities (karmic baggage and external projections), and it can't be resolved by yelling, screaming, crying, or letting the emotion rise through your energy system to the organs of expression in your face. It's worth noting that just because an emotion is inauthentic doesn't mean you won't feel it.

## Space and the Resolution of Emotions

The time it takes for your authentic emotions to be expressed provides you with the space you need for creative ideas to evolve into a form that you can manifest successfully in the world. Space is closely connected to the condition of your auric fields and the quality of energy contained within them.

Auric fields are large fields of prana that fill and surround your subtle energy field on each dimension. From the surface of your body on each dimension, your auric fields extend outward (in all directions) from about two inches (six centimeters) to more than twenty-six feet (almost eight meters). Refer back to Figure 7.

Structurally, each auric field is composed of an inner cavity and a thin surface boundary that surrounds it and gives it its characteristic egg shape. Functionally, each auric field serves as both a reservoir of prana and a boundary that separates your internal environment from the external environment.

To recover your inner voice, your auras on each dimension must be strong, firm, and free from the inordinate accumulation of karmic baggage.

Your second task will be to fill your auric fields surrounding your first through sixth chakras with prana so that there is more space, and therefore more time, for your authentic emotions to be expressed.

---

### Exercise: Filling Auric Fields with Prana

To fill your auric fields with prana, find a comfortable position with your back straight. Breathe deeply through your nose for two to three minutes. Then count backward from five to one and from ten to one. Use the Standard Method to relax your muscles and to center yourself in your authentic mind. Then assert, *"It's my intent to center myself in my prakriti field."* Next, you will fill your auric fields on the first through sixth dimensions with prana. To do that, assert, *"It's my intent to fill the auric fields surrounding my first through sixth chakras with prana."* Don't do anything after that—just enjoy the process for the next fifteen minutes.

After fifteen minutes, count from one to five. Then open your eyes and bring yourself out of the meditation. Repeat as needed.

### The Third Task

Your next task will be to enhance your sensuality. To do that, you must enhance the sensitivity of your organs of perception. You may not be aware of it, but your ability to sense worldly things through your organs of perception—sight, hearing, taste, smell, and touch—is regulated by the organs of your energy field, particularly your chakras. Therefore, it should come as no surprise that, if you activate the appropriate chakras, you can enhance the function of your senses. That in turn will enhance your sensuality and help liberate your inner voice.

In the exercise that follows, you will use the chakras in your body space along with the corresponding chakras below body space to enhance your sense of touch, taste, smell, sight, and hearing.

Before we proceed, we will examine the first six chakras below personal space because, along with your seven traditional chakras, they have the most impact on your organs of perception and your ability to sense worldly things.

The chakras below body space begin their descent just below your first chakra at the base of your spine. The first chakra below body space is located about two-and-a-half inches (six centimeters) below the perineum, and the remaining chakras extend downward for approximately twenty feet (six meters) (see Figure 7).

If you study Figure 7, you'll see that the chakras below personal body space are almost identical to the chakras within body space, except for their length. They are about 40 percent shorter.

In the exercise that follows, you will enhance the functions of your organs of perception by activating the appropriate chakra in body space and the corresponding chakra below it. After you've activated the appropriate chakras, you will center yourself in the chakra fields on the dimensions regulated by the two chakras you've activated.

To enhance your sense of touch, you will activate your third chakra and your third chakra below body space. Then you will center yourself in both chakra fields. To enhance your sense of smell and taste, you will activate your fifth chakra and your fifth chakra below personal body space. Then you will center yourself in both chakra fields. To enhance your sense of sight and hearing, you will activate your sixth chakra and your sixth chakra below personal body space. Then you will center yourself in both chakra fields.

You will perform the exercise by enhancing your sense of touch. Afterward, you can use the same technique to enhance the function of your other senses by activating the appropriate chakras and centering yourself in their corresponding chakra fields.

---

## Exercise: Enhancing Sensuality

To enhance your sense of touch, find a comfortable position with your back straight. Close your eyes and breathe deeply through your nose for two to three minutes. Then count backward from five to one and from ten to one. Use the Standard Method to relax your muscles and to center yourself in your authentic mind. Then assert, *"It's my intent to activate my third chakra."* Continue by asserting, *"It's my intent to activate my third chakra below body space."* Take a few moments to enjoy the shift. Then assert, *"It's my intent to center myself in my third chakra field."* Next, assert, *"It's my intent to center myself in the third chakra field below my body space."* Continue by asserting, *"It's my intent to turn my organs of perception inward on the levels of my third chakra and third chakra below body space."*

Take fifteen minutes to enjoy the experience. Then count from one to five and bring yourself out of the meditation. Repeat as needed

### The Fourth Task: Reclaiming Your Inner Voice

Now, that you've made all the necessary preparations, you're ready to reclaim your inner voice by performing the Inner Voice Mudra.

To perform the mudra, sit in a comfortable position with your back straight. Use the Standard Method to relax your muscles and to center yourself in your authentic mind. Then bring the tip of your tongue to your upper palate and hold it at the point where the back of your teeth meet your gum. Put the tips of your pinkies together next so that they form a triangle. Continue by putting the outside of your ring fingers together so that they're touching one another from first to second joint.

Put the tips of your middle fingers together to form a second triangle. Then bring the outside of your index fingers together so that they're touching from the first to second joint. Finally, overlap your thumbs so that the tips of your thumbs are touching your index fingers at a point between the second joints and your knuckles

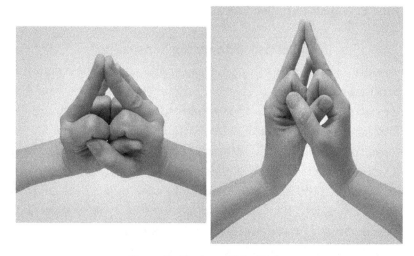

*Figure 13: The Inner Voice Mudra*

Hold the mudra for ten minutes and enjoy the shift as your inner voice emerges and your creative juices once again flow freely. After ten minutes, release the mudra. Then count from one to five and bring yourself out of the exercise.

By performing all four tasks for as little as two weeks, you will reclaim your inner voice. And once again, you will be able to manifest your creativity in the world. Repeat as needed.

## Summary

In this chapter, you learned to enhance your creativity by performing the Purusha Field Meditation and by restoring your inner voice. In the next chapter you will learn how you can increase your inner beauty, regardless of your age, so that it transforms the way you look and how other people perceive you.

We've included tips on how to use food, exercise, natural environments, negative ions, and beautiful things to enhance your inner beauty and radiance. Special attention has been given to good character and its influence on female radiance. To enhance good character when necessary, we've included a series of easy to perform exercises.

## NINE
# Enhancing Female Radiance

### Inner Beauty

Inner beauty is a form of radiance that emerges from deep within a woman's energy field. It changes how a woman feels about herself. And it changes how people perceive her. In this chapter, we will attempt to cut through the rubbish that panders to the insecurities of women and get to the basic truth about inner beauty—what it is and what it is not. Then we will look into how a woman can increase her inner beauty, regardless of her age, so that it will not only transform the way she looks, it will transform how other people perceive her.

In most people's minds, beauty is connected exclusively with a woman's physical features. But there are people who already recognize that beauty is dependent on how a person feels. A woman can have perfect features and a youthful, athletic body. But if she doesn't feel good, if she is depressed, stressed or exhausted, or lacks self-esteem or character, or is conflicted and can't radiate her energy freely, even if she has all the assets associated with physical beauty she won't feel beautiful, and she won't be considered beautiful by other people.

On the other hand, good character, a healthy body, and an abundance of feminine energy can make any woman look beautiful, even if she doesn't have perfect features. Such a woman will gain the respect and admiration of the people she knows because she will radiate the glow associated with a beautiful woman. It's this glow that is the foundation of beauty. And it's this glow that will make a woman feel beautiful when she looks at herself in the mirror and when she looks into the eyes of other people.

## The Inner Glow

You may not be aware of it, but everything we see in the external environment is an interpretation of the world around us. We never see the world as it actually is because of the limitations of our organs of perception and the way we interpret our experiences.

When someone we perceive gives us a bad feeling, even if they have perfect features, they can appear ugly. And when someone we perceive gives us a good feeling, even if they have imperfect features, they can appear beautiful. So, when we deal with beauty, we're not simply dealing with bone structure and flawless skin; we're dealing with appearances that are subjective.

It's also useful to remember that physical beauty can become a burden, or in extreme cases, a deficit. We've all heard stories about women who were taken advantage of or marginalized at work because of their beauty. In contrast, inner beauty always enhances a woman's life, regardless of what the propagandists in the media tell us.

## Enhancing Inner Beauty

So, what enhances inner beauty? From our work, we've learned that inner beauty has four essential aspects: good health, character, inner peace, and feminine energy.

## Good Health

Inner beauty has always been associated with good health. When we talk about health, we're talking about both physical health and the health of a woman's subtle energy field.

Physical activities that disrupt good health include smoking, drinking alcohol, and doing drugs to excess. Inactivity, as well as stressful mental activities such as worrying also interfere with good health. All of these activities disrupt good health by interfering with the flow of prana and by disrupting the energetic balance between a woman's physical body and subtle energy field.

Promoting good health and inner beauty therefore means less smoking, less drinking, fewer drugs, and a less sedentary lifestyle. It also means that you must get more natural. You have a physical body that is designed to interact with the natural environment. And even though life in the twenty-first century may force you to spend long periods of time in man-made environments, it's natural things that have the most positive effect on your health and well-being.

Food is one natural thing that promotes good health. You may be forced to work in an office building and drive a car on the highway to and from work, but no one forces you to eat processed foods that provide empty calories but little else. Experience has taught us that food has an immense effect on beauty and good health. Fresh foods that are natural and not adulterated have the most life-affirming qualities. They protect you against free radicals and other toxic substances. And they contain vitamins and nutrients that will keep your metabolism healthy. Fresh foods also have nutrients that can reduce stress, keep your muscles firm, and your skin soft and subtle.

We've listed several foods that you can add to your diet. Each has beneficial properties that promote inner beauty and good health.

**Mangos:** have carotene, which protects a woman from UV damage and enhances the radiance of a woman's skin. They contain zinc, which improves the strength and luster of your hair. Mangos improve the health of the gums and tighten your connective tissue. They're rich in vitamin A, which enhances vitality, and they have mood enhancing properties. Eating mangos can actually make you feel euphoric.

**Papayas:** contain large amounts of vitamin A, which will improve vision and give your eyes a healthy glow. They enhance the function of enzymes that promote vitality and other essential life processes. Papayas improve the functions of your heart and circulation. And they enhance the function of your colon, which will enhance the health of your skin and improve your muscle tone.

**Cherries:** contain folic acid, which improves cell metabolism. Folic acid is one of the most important vitamins a woman can take during pregnancy because it plays a prominent role in the production of nerve cells. Cherries also contain large amounts of iron that has rejuvenating properties that promote healthy gums and skin.

**Saffron:** has aphrodisiacal and regenerative properties. In Ayurvedic medicine, saffron has been used to fight depression and to harmonize and balance a woman's menstrual cycle.

**Garlic:** known for its rejuvenating and regenerating properties. Garlic can lower a woman's cholesterol level and help her body discharge metabolic waste. It's good for the heart and can be used to fight infections, skin diseases, and sciatic problems.

### Avoid Eating at Night

Although fresh, healthy foods enhance inner beauty, eating too much, or eating late at night, can have a negative influence on health and radiance.

Eating at night will add pounds to your body because nighttime metabolism is incomplete. In addition, your body is rebuilding cells while you're sleeping. If you eat late at night, your body must perform this essential task along with the difficult work of digestion. This stresses your body by increasing your blood pressure, increasing the production of LDL cholesterol, and increasing blood sugar, all of which are risk factors for diabetes and other diseases. In Europe, an old proverb states, "Frühstücken wie ein Kaiser, Mittagessen wie ein König, und Abendessen wie ein Bettler" (Eat breakfast like an emperor, lunch like a king, and dinner like a beggar).

### Physical Exercise

Exercise enhances female radiance in a host of ways. It enhances muscle tone and increases mental alertness. By improving blood circulation, it helps release toxins that are responsible for aging. Exercise improves sleep, which has its own health and beauty benefits, and it enhances the production of serotonin, which enhances pleasure and helps a woman overcome the effects of depression.

Strenuous, regular exercise will help you transcend your limitations, which in turn will help you overcome fear and anxiety. Stress hormones will be reduced when you exercise regularly, and so will physical tension.

For those of you looking for a regular regimen of physical exercise, we recommend Hatha Yoga or Tai Chi. These forms of exercise not only provide health benefits, they help to integrate the activities of your physical body with the activities of your subtle energy field.

### Natural Environments

Good health and natural environments go hand in hand. Natural environments, especially forests, have a rejuvenating effect on people. But not all forests are the same. Old growth forests are renowned for their ecological complexity and the age of their trees. Less appreciated is the fact that old trees radiate vast amounts of prana into the environment. When there are a number of old trees growing together, the atmosphere around them will be saturated with prana. The effect can be so pronounced that depression can be lifted and anxiety reduced. The enhanced radiation of prana and the pleasure it brings will benefit women physically and energetically by enhancing their ability to connect to the earth and to other people.

Almost all national forests in the U.S. and Canada have groves of old growth, especially at higher elevations. Take a hike, take friends, and take some natural, fresh food along for a picnic.

### Enjoy Beautiful Things

When a woman enjoys beautiful things—art, nature, and beautiful man-made objects—pupils widen and there is an emotional reaction. Music can have a particularly positive effect on a woman's beauty and health. The complexity of certain types of music stimulates parts of the brain linked to creativity, concentration, and abstract thinking.

It isn't well-known, but the seven tones in the major musical scale are linked energetically to the seven traditional chakras. Baroque composers, and even some modern composers, were aware of this connection and created music that stimulated the chakras, and simultaneously provided listeners with an endorphin rush.

### Negative Ions

Negative ions are created in nature as air molecules break apart due to sunlight, moving air, and water. They're odorless, tasteless, and invisible molecules that we inhale in abundance in certain environments. Think mountains, waterfalls, and beaches. Once they reach our bloodstream, negative ions are believed to produce biochemical reactions that increase levels of the mood-enhancing chemical serotonin. It's believed that enhanced serotonin levels help alleviate depression, relieve stress, and boost energy—all of which enhance health and beauty.

Fortunately, every home has a built in natural ionizer: the shower. We suggest that you give yourself a negative ion bath by spraying your body with cold water from the showerhead at least once a day.

## Good Character

Energy with universal qualities is both the foundation and product of good character. This means that women who have self-discipline and patience as well as courage and who persevere in what they do radiate prana freely and glow with inner beauty. On the other hand, if a woman is trapped in distorted energy and is undisciplined, if she is intolerant of other people's defects and is unreliable because she doesn't persevere or have the courage to live with integrity, then she will have very little prana available. As a result, she will become stiff and her posture will suffer. Her eyes will become dull and instead of moving with grace and radiating feminine qualities freely, she will become self-conscious and sullen because of the distorted energy that dominates her subtle energetic interactions.

Of course, all this can be avoided if a woman chooses to enhance her good character. With this in mind, we've included an exercise for each quality associated with good character. So, instead of dwelling on your character defects, practice the exercises we've provided, and in a short time you will receive the benefits, which include the inner beauty and radiance that come from having good character.

## Patience

To enhance your patience, you will perform the Patience Mudra. To begin, sit in a comfortable position with your back straight. Use the Standard Method to relax and to center yourself in your authentic mind. Then bring the tip of your tongue to the point where your gums and upper teeth meet. Put the soles of your feet together next. Then cup your hands together tightly while you press your left thumb against the outside of your right pinky and your right thumb against the outside of your right index finger. Hold for ten minutes with your eyes closed. Repeat as needed.

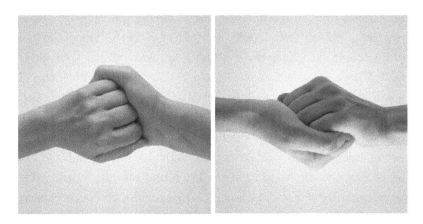

*Figure 14: The Patience Mudra*

## Perseverance

People can't persevere when they don't have enough prana. To enhance your perseverance, you will increase the pressure in your energy field. That in turn will enhance the amount of prana flowing through it. The simplest way to increase the pressure in your energy field is to activate your first and seventh chakras, center yourself in the corresponding chakra fields, and use your intent to enhance the flow of prana through your governor meridian. To do that, close your eyes and breathe deeply through your nose for two to three minutes. Then count backward from five to one and from ten to one. Use the Standard Method to relax your muscles and to center yourself in your authentic mind. Then assert, *"It's my intent to activate my first chakra."* Next, assert, *"It's my intent to center myself in my first chakra field."* Continue by asserting, *"It's my intent to activate my seventh chakra."* Next, assert, *"It's my intent to center myself in my seventh chakra field."* To complete the exercise, assert, *"It's my intent increase the flow of prana through my governor meridian."* Take ten minutes to enjoy the effects. Then count from one to five and open your eyes. If you practice the exercise for as little as a week, there will be a noticeable increase in your perseverance. Repeat as needed.

### Non-harming

In order to overcome distorted fields of energy that support harmful thoughts, feelings, and actions, you must be able to empathize with other people. You have three fields of empathy within your energy field. They are resource fields that supply your chakras with energy. To overcome the tendency to harm other people, you will fill these fields with prana and radiate the excess energy through your etheric chakras.

To begin, close your eyes and breathe deeply through your nose for two to three minutes. Then count backward from five to one and from ten to one. Use the Standard Method to relax your muscles and to center yourself in your authentic mind. Then assert, *"It's my intent to activate my upper etheric chakra."* Continue by asserting, *"It's my intent to activate my lower etheric chakra."* Next, assert, *"It's my intent to center myself in my three fields of empathy."*

Once you're centered in your three fields of empathy, assert, *"It's my intent to fill my three fields of empathy with prana."* Then assert, *"It's my intent to radiate prana from my three fields of empathy through my etheric chakras."* Enjoy the effects for fifteen minutes. Then count from one to five and bring yourself out of the meditation. Repeat as needed.

### Discipline

Problems with discipline are directly related to polarity problems in your subtle energy field. Although it appears that there are two fields of polarity, once you enter the non-physical universe, you will encounter additional fields of polarity that influence your energetic interactions. When it comes to discipline, it's the third polar field, the neutral field, which is most important.

By centering yourself in your third polar field, you will free yourself from the push and pull of distorted energy fields. And you will be able to remain focused and disciplined in a chaotic and ever changing world.

To enhance discipline, close your eyes and breathe deeply through your nose for two to three minutes. Then count backward from five to one and from ten to one. Use the Standard Method to relax your muscles and to center yourself in your authentic mind. Then assert, *"It's my intent to center myself in my third polar field."* Next, assert, *"It's my intent to turn my organs of perception inward in my third polar field."* Stay centered for fifteen minutes. Then count from one to five and bring yourself out of the meditation. Repeat as needed.

### Long-suffering

This is the ability to remain steadfast when times are turbulent and/or difficult. In order to remain steadfast, you must enhance your ability to experience joy and manifest it in the world. Your second chakra regulates sexual joy. Your fifth chakra regulates unconditional joy. To enhance long-suffering, you will activate your second and fifth chakras and center yourself in their corresponding chakra fields. Then you will activate the minor energy centers in your hands and feet.

To begin, close your eyes and breathe deeply through your nose for two to three minutes. Then count backward from five to one and from ten to one. Use the Standard Method to relax your muscles and to center yourself in your authentic mind. Then assert, *"It's my intent to activate my second chakra."* Continue by asserting, *"It's my intent to activate my fifth chakra."* After the two chakras are active, assert, *"It's my intent to center myself in my second chakra field."* Continue by asserting, *"It's my intent to center myself in my fifth chakra field."*

Take a few moments to enjoy the shift. Then assert, *"It's my intent to activate the minor energy centers in my hands."* Continue by asserting, *"It's my intent to activate the minor energy centers in my feet."* Stay centered for fifteen minutes. Then count from one to five and bring yourself out of the meditation.

If you practice the exercise regularly, you will remain steadfast and self-confident even when times are difficult. Repeat as needed.

### Courage

Courage is a feeling that is associated with the kidneys. Your third chakra regulates the prana in the section of your body that includes your kidneys. When your third chakra is blocked and subtle energy can't radiate through your kidneys, you will experience fear. Without the contraction caused by fear, both physical and moral courage will emerge spontaneously.

In order to enhance your courage, you will perform the Enhanced Courage Meditation. To begin, find a comfortable position with your back straight. Breathe deeply through your nose for two to three minutes. Then count backward from five to one and from ten to one. Use the Standard Method to relax your muscles and to center yourself in your authentic mind. Then assert, *"It's my intent to active my third chakra."* Next, assert, *"It's my intent to center myself in my third chakra field."* Continue by asserting, *"It's my intent to fill my third chakra field with prana."* Take a few moments to enjoy the shift. Then assert, *"It's my intent to activate the minor energy centers in my hands."* As soon as your minor energy centers are active, place one palm on each of your kidneys. By doing that you will enhance the flow of prana through your kidneys. That in turn will enhance the feelings associated with courage.

Continue for fifteen minutes. Then remove your hands, count from one to five, and bring yourself out of the meditation. Repeat as needed.

## Feminine Energy

Feminine energy, in the form of prana, is so powerful that, when a woman radiates it freely, people will be captivated by the inner glow that permeates her body and mind. In order to enhance the amount of feminine energy radiating through your subtle energy field—so that the inner glow transforms you and the way you look—you will perform the Prakriti Field Meditation.

The field of prakriti is a resource field that contains some of the highest and purest frequencies of feminine energy. Like all resource fields, the prakriti field fills your energy field and extends beyond it in all directions. By centering yourself in the prakriti field, you will experience primordial feminine energy. This is the energy that creates and sustains life and provides you with the strength to become a radiant woman.

## Exercise: The Prakriti Field Meditation

To begin the meditation, find a comfortable position with your back straight. Close your eyes and breathe deeply through your nose for two to three minutes. Then count backward from five to one and from ten to one. Use the Standard Method to relax your muscles and to center yourself in your authentic mind. Then assert, *"It's my intent to center myself in my prakriti field."* Continue by asserting, *"It's my intent to turn my organs of perception inward in my prakriti field."* After a few moments, your orientation will shift and you'll become aware of a large cavity that fills your physical body and extends beyond it. This cavity is the prakriti field.

From your new vantage point within the field of prakriti you will become aware of feminine power and love in its primordial form. And you will feel them both radiating through you freely.

Take fifteen minutes to enjoy the experience. Then count from one to five. When you reach the number five, open your eyes and bring yourself out of the meditation. Repeat as needed.

The more often you practice the Prakriti Field Meditation, the greater the benefits will be and the easier it will be to experience the radiance that comes from the universal feminine within you.

## Inner Peace

Inner peace is a state of stillness that emerges from deep within you. It emerges when movement stops and you can focus your mind on the joy that spontaneously radiates through your energy field. The Inner Peace Mudra is designed to help you experience inner peace regardless of your personal circumstances.

To perform the Inner Peace Mudra, sit in a comfortable position with your back straight. Use the Standard Method to relax your muscles and to center yourself in your authentic mind. Then place your left thumb on the acupuncture point on the inside edge of your right thumb, just below the nail. Place the inside tips of your index fingers together. Your middle fingers are curved inward and touching from the first to second joint. The pads of your ring fingers are touching up to the first joint. And your left pinkie is placed over the nail of your right pinkie from the tip to the first joint.

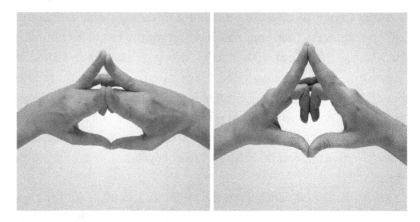

*Figure 15: The Inner Peace Mudra*

Keep the soles of your feet flat on the floor and your tongue in its normal position. Hold the mudra for ten minutes with your eyes closed. After ten minutes, count from one to five and open your eyes. Repeat as needed.

## Summary

In this chapter, you learned that a woman can enhance her inner beauty by enhancing her health and character, by experiencing greater inner peace, and by enhancing the flow of prana through her energy field. In the next chapter, you will learn how to overcome the chronic and acute symptoms of trauma. Special attention has been given to past life trauma, physical and psychological trauma, sexual trauma, and to the trauma of neglect.

# TEN

# Healing Traumas to Your Body, Soul, and Spirit

We will begin this chapter by looking at how a traumatic event can cripple a woman on both the physical and subtle energetic levels. After that, you will learn to perform three exercises designed to heal the energetic wounds that are responsible for their most enduring symptoms. Then we will provide you with exercises and tips designed to permanently overcome the patterns and psychological symptoms caused by the most common traumas modern women must endure: past life trauma, physical and psychological trauma, sexual trauma, and the trauma of neglect.

## Trauma, the Inside Story

Although medical and mental health practitioners have studied the various forms of trauma for years, they still have trouble defining them. That's because it's almost impossible to define or even describe a traumatic event without taking into consideration the violence done to the survivor's subtle energy field. There is a simple reason for this: it's the violence done to the subtle energy field that is responsible for the most acute and enduring symptoms the survivor must endure.

To understand why a traumatic event can have a long-term effect on a person, it's important to recognize that every traumatic event is really a dual event that includes two traumas, a physical-psychological trauma and a subtle energetic trauma that is non-physical, but no less real.

Memory of the physical and psychological trauma may be repressed, but the energetic trauma will continue to emerge into the survivor's consciousness for years as a disruption of authentic identity and gender orientation. It will also contribute to the breakdown of the survivor's trust, which will disrupt self-esteem and make it difficult for the survivor to participate in long-term, intimate relationships.

From our experience, we've learned that an energetic trauma will have three significant effects on the survivor. There will be a violent intrusion of distorted energy into the survivor's energy field. The violence of the energetic intrusion will cause one or more energetic vehicles to be ejected. This is known as "fragmentation." And, the intrusion will disrupt the flow of prana though the survivor's subtle energy system. It's these three energetic affects that create lifelong problems for the survivor, problems that cannot normally be corrected by conventional therapy or orthodox medicine.

## Second Generation Symptoms

Even though an energetic trauma will have an immediate effect on the survivor's subtle energy field, most people who've been traumatized won't recognize the first generation symptoms. Only later, when the second and third generation symptoms emerge, will most people recognize that something is seriously wrong. Second generation symptoms include the disruption of self-control, trust, personal power, self-esteem, and vitality. Depression and anxiety are common second generation symptoms.

As time passes, these energetic and psychological symptoms can lead to a loss of motivation, sexual dysfunction, creative blocks, and boundary problems that can cause the survivor to withdraw from the normal activities of everyday life.

When it's a child who is traumatized, there will be additional long-term complications. These include a disruption of personal identity and the creation of blind spots, which will make it difficult for the child to succeed in school and form healthy relationships with other children. Blind spots are created when the pain and fear are too difficult to bear and the child pushes the event as well as portions of their mind and subtle energy field out of conscious awareness. When this happens, the child will lose access to the functions of mind trapped within these blind spots. This means that portions of the mind and subtle energy field can no longer be used to interact with other people in healthy ways. As a result, the survivor can become rigid, unyielding, and unable to empathize or even understand the views and feelings of others.

Since the three energetic wounds described above are responsible for the most enduring symptoms that traumas produce, you will learn to overcome them first. After that we will provide you with a series of exercises designed specifically to heal the second-generation symptoms caused by the most common traumas that children, young girls, and women experience.

Since it's the intrusion of distorted energy into the survivor's subtle energy field that is responsible for all subsequent symptoms, you will learn to heal intrusions first.

## Intrusions

An intrusion is created by the violent projection of distorted energy into the survivor's subtle energy field. If you are the target of an intrusion, you may feel like a pin or dart has punctured your skin when it makes contact with your subtle energy field. The intrusion may also make you feel like you're being smothered, or that a wave of discordant energy is pouring into you.

You don't have to be in physical contact with the perpetrator to be the target of an intrusion. People who are attached to dense fields of energy can project them into your subtle energy field when they think about you, have strong feelings about you, or have the desire to change, manipulate, control, or punish you.

---

### Exercise: Releasing Intrusions

Fortunately, with the knowledge and skills you've already acquired, you have all the tools necessary to release an intrusion of distorted energy from your subtle energy field. In fact, releasing an intrusion is no more difficult than releasing karmic baggage. The first step will be to choose a feeling, attitude, blockage, or self-limiting pattern that creates an irrational fear of a particular person, place, or thing, or that consistently interferes with your ability to be yourself, express yourself freely, and achieve your goals.

Examples of feelings caused by intrusions are panic, foreboding, rage, frustration, anxiety, alienation, arrogance, contempt, chronic irritation, and annoyance. Examples of patterns caused by intrusions include self-doubt, self-sabotage, helplessness, despondency, dependency, insecurity, indolence, and a lack of self-worth.

Once you've chosen a pattern or feeling to work on, find a comfortable position with your back straight. Then close your eyes and breathe deeply through your nose for two to three minutes. Use the Standard Method to relax your muscles and to center yourself in your authentic mind. Then perform the Orgasmic Bliss Mudra (go to chapter 4) and continue to hold it while you assert, *"It's my intent to create a prana box around the intrusion that causes the (your feeling or pattern here) I have in mind."* Once you can see and/or sense the prana box, continue by asserting, *"It's my intent to fill the prana box I created with bliss."* Then assert, *"It's my intent that bliss releases the intrusion in my prana box."*

As soon as the intrusion has been released, there will be a sense of relief, which is often accompanied by a pop that indicates that the only thing that remains in your prana box is bliss.

Once you've released the intrusion, release the prana box. Then release the Orgasmic Bliss Mudra. Take ten minutes to enjoy the changes you experience. Then count from one to five and bring yourself out of the meditation.

## Fragmentation

Your energy field will become fragmented whenever an energetic vehicle has been ejected from it. The most common cause of fragmentation is the intrusion of distorted energy into your energy field. Fragmentation can take place on any dimension, during any phase of a person's life, including the nine months between conception and birth. Fragmentation and its collateral effects has become so common that overcoming fragmentation by decontaminating and reintegrating energetic vehicles has become an essential part of healing and energy work. That's because energetic vehicles carry out a host of vital functions. They allow you to form an authentic identity and to interact with your environment on both the physical and non-physical levels. Energetic vehicles also help you to manifest your soul urge and fulfill your dharma.

To heal fragmentation you must first locate an energetic vehicle that has been ejected. Then you must decontaminate it and reintegrate it into your energy field.

To locate an energetic vehicle that has been ejected from your energy field and decontaminate it, you will use the same technique used to locate and release karmic baggage in chapter 4.

Once you've located and decontaminated an energetic vehicle, you must reintegrate it so that it's congruent. For an energetic vehicle to be congruent, it must be centered exactly in the middle of your body space. Congruence is important for several reasons. It permits the reintegrated vehicle to function synchronistically with other energetic vehicles in your energy field. It facilitates the uninterrupted flow of prana through it. And it allows you to reintegrate it into your authentic identity.

## Exercise: Healing Fragmentation

To heal fragmentation, find a comfortable position with your back straight. Then close your eyes and breathe deeply through your nose for two to three minutes. Use the Standard Method to relax your muscles and to center yourself in your authentic mind. Then perform the Orgasmic Bliss Mudra and hold it. Next, assert, *"It's my intent to create a prana box around my energetic vehicle that has been ejected furthest from body space by the intrusion I released in the last exercise."* Continue by asserting, *"It's my intent to fill the prana box I just created with bliss and to reintegrate the energetic vehicle within it into my subtle energy field."* Don't do anything after that. Your energetic vehicle will be decontaminated and reintegrated automatically. After the energetic vehicle has become congruent, take ten minutes to enjoy the effects. Then release the prana box, the Orgasmic Bliss Mudra, and bring yourself out of the meditation by counting from one to five.

Once congruence has been achieved, you will experience a sense of satisfaction, greater inner strength, and stability.

Since a traumatic experience can cause more than one energetic vehicle to be ejected, you may have to repeat the process more than once. To do that, always reintegrate the energetic vehicle that is farthest from your energy field first. In this way you will consistently reintegrate all the energetic vehicles that were ejected as a result of a traumatic experience.

Mistakes are inevitable. This means that you may reintegrate an energetic vehicle that still contains contaminants. If you do, symptoms will emerge almost immediately. The most common symptoms will be sudden anti-self and anti-social feelings, which emerge from contaminants within the energetic vehicle. To correct the situation, you will have to remove the contaminants (while the energetic vehicle is in your energy field).

The process is essentially the same one you used to release karmic baggage. Simply use your intent and mental attention to place the energetic vehicle in a prana box. Perform the Orgasmic Bliss Mudra and hold it while you assert, *"It's my intent that bliss fills the prana box I just created and releases all the contaminants in it."* Bliss will release any residual contamination—and it will also assure that the energetic vehicle is properly integrated.

## Restoring the Flow of Prana

Whenever you experience a traumatic event, the flow of prana through your energy field will be disrupted. The energetic flow will be partially restored once you've removed the intrusions responsible for the trauma and reintegrated your energetic vehicles that have been ejected. However, to fully restore the flow of prana to healthy levels, you must reactivate your thirteen chakras in body space as well as the first six above it.

---

## Exercise: Activating the
## First through Thirteenth Chakras

To restore the flow of prana through your energy field, find a comfortable position with your back straight. Then close your eyes and breathe deeply through your nose for two to three minutes. After two to three minutes, count backward from five to one then ten to one. Use the Standard Method to relax your muscles and to center yourself in your authentic mind. Then assert, *"It's my intent to activate my first chakra."* Next, assert, *"It's my intent to center myself in my first chakra field."* Continue in the same way by activating your second, third, fourth, fifth, sixth, and seventh traditional chakras, and by centering yourself in the corresponding chakra fields. Continue in the same way with the upper and lower physical chakras and the upper and lower physical-material chakras.

Take a few moments to enjoy the affects. Then activate your eighth, ninth, tenth, eleventh, twelfth, and thirteenth chakras above body space, and center yourself in the corresponding chakra fields. After you've activated all thirteen chakras and centered yourself in all thirteen chakra fields in body space and the first six above body space, assert, *"On the levels of my first through thirteenth chakras in body space and the first six above body space, it's my intent to turn my organs of perception inward."* Finally, assert, *"It's my intent to fill my chakra fields on the first through thirteenth dimensions and the next six above my head with prana."*

Take fifteen minutes to enjoy the changes you experience. Then count from one to five. When you reach the number five open your eyes. You will feel wide-awake, perfectly relaxed, and better than you did before. By practicing this exercise regularly, you will restore the flow of prana through your chakras and chakra fields. This will enable you to overcome many of the residual effects that are the legacy of the traumatic event you experienced.

## Healing a Past Life Trauma

Now that you've learned to heal the first generation energetic symptoms created by a traumatic event, we will examine the four most common traumas people experience in the modern world: past life trauma, physical and psychological trauma, the trauma of neglect, and sexual trauma. We will begin by examining past life trauma.

Like karmic baggage, past life traumas can make it difficult for you to establish a healthy identity, form intimate relationships, fulfill your dharma, and experience your power, creativity, and radiance. In addition, they can create self-limiting patterns that make subsequent wounds and traumas almost inevitable.

Although it's quite common to have past life traumas linked to self-limiting patterns and traumatic events in this life, healing a past life trauma is no more difficult than healing any other energetic wound. However, to heal a past life trauma, it's essential to connect the events that took place in your past life to the self-limiting patterns and traumatic events you experienced in this life. To do that, you will learn to perform the Silver Cord Meditation. Each energy body is connected to the energy field of a person by a silver cord that extends from the back of the neck and can stretch almost indefinitely.

---

### Exercise: Silver Cord Meditation

To perform the Silver Cord Meditation, choose a feeling, attitude, blockage, or self-limiting pattern that you've had since you were a child. It should be something that has consistently interfered with your ability to be yourself, follow your dharma, and to feel and express yourself freely. Once you've made your choice, find a comfortable position with your back straight. Then count backward from ten to one and then five to one. Use the Standard Method to relax your muscles and to center yourself in your authentic mind. Then assert, *"It's my intent to create the visual screen eight feet (two-and-a-half meters) in front of me."* Once the screen appears, assert, *"It's my intent to follow a silver cord from the back of my neck to the traumatic event I've chosen to heal—and to view the event on the screen in front of me."* Don't do anything after that.

Let yourself get drawn into this past life drama that caused the trauma. Stay alert and don't ignore any quality that emerges into your conscious awareness: feelings, sounds, the physical environment, and the actions and expressions of people. Everything that you see on the screen or feel in your body and energy field will provide you with valuable details.

Once you've re-experienced the events that led to the trauma on both the physical and non-physical levels, release the images on the screen. Then release the screen and count from one to five to bring yourself out of the meditation.

It's a good idea to write down what you experienced in the Silver Cord Meditation and to remain receptive to additional insights that emerge into your conscious awareness.

When you're ready to proceed, use the three exercises you learned earlier in this chapter to release the intrusions that connect you to the perpetrator, to decontaminate and reintegrate the energetic vehicles that were ejected from your energy field because of fragmentation, and to restore the flow of prana through your energy field. Repeat the exercises as needed.

## Healing Physical and Psychological Trauma

We've put physical and psychological trauma in one category because, in both cases, the energetic violation will be virtually the same. In both cases, there will be a sustained attack that will break down the survivor's natural defenses.

If the target of an attack can successfully defend herself or himself physically and energetically, the violence may be extreme, and even sustained, but the survivor won't be traumatized. A good example is childhood fights that can cause physical injury and emotional distress but have no long-term energetic affect.

To overcome the effects of physical and/or psychological trauma, you must restore the health of your energy field as well as your courage. To do that, you will use the exercises you learned earlier in this chapter to release intrusions, to overcome fragmentation, and to restore the flow of prana through your energy field. After that, you will restore your courage by performing the Core Field Meditation.

---

### Exercise: The Core Field Meditation

To begin the Core Field Meditation, find a comfortable position with your back straight. Then close your eyes and breathe deeply through your nose for two to three minutes. Use the Standard Method to relax your muscles and to center yourself in your authentic mind. Then assert, *"It's my intent to center myself in my core field."* Continue by asserting, *"It's my intent to turn my organs of perception inward on the level of my core field."* Take a few moments to enjoy the shift. Then assert, *"It's my intent to fill my core field with prana in the section associated with courage."* Take fifteen minutes to experience the shift in your level of courage and self-confidence. Then count from one to five and bring yourself out of the meditation. Repeat as needed.

## Healing the Trauma of Neglect

One type of trauma that is often overlooked by medical practitioners is neglect. A woman can experience the trauma of neglect if her parents or guardians don't want her, if they want a boy, or if they're too self-involved to care for her properly. Neglect always involves the rejection of the child psychologically and energetically. That's because the neglectful adult will project distorted energy from their karmic baggage at the child in an effort to push her away. As with all traumatic events, the violent projection of distorted energy will create an intrusion. That in turn will cause fragmentation and disrupt the flow of prana through the child's energy field.

Although no two women have the same experience as a child or adolescent, there are some elements of neglect that are universal. Neglect produces feelings of abandonment and isolation. It disrupts trust. And it makes the formation of a life-affirming identity difficult.

To overcome the effects of neglect, we've provided you with a five-part program. The program is followed by a two-day pause, and repeated until recovery is complete.

### Day 1

On day one, you will release the intrusion that was used by the neglectful adult to push you away. Then you will reintegrate the energetic vehicles that were ejected from your energy field. After that you will enhance the flow of prana through your energy field by activating the thirteen chakras in body space and the first six above body space.

### Day 2

On day two, you will activate your first and third chakras and center yourself in your first and third chakra fields (go to chapter 3).

*Day 3*

On day three, you will perform the Trust and Self-Esteem Mudras (go to chapter 2 and chapter 5).

*Day 4*

On day four, you will use the visual screen to create an archetype that fosters self-confidence and stability. We suggest you use the archetype of the innocent woman (go to chapter 5).

*Day 5*

On day five, you will enhance your connection to the universal feminine by performing the Precious Jewel Mudra (go to chapter 1).

## Sexual Trauma

Contrary to what many people think, sexual abuse is not exclusively about sex. Sexual abuse comes in many forms, but regardless of the form it takes, sexual abuse is fundamentally about power and control.

Although we're all familiar with the overt forms of sexual abuse, in Western society the subtle forms of sexual abuse are often overlooked. This means that many people who've been sexually abused, particularly as children, fail to recognize the extent of the energetic trauma they experienced. In addition, they may not recognize that the effects of the abuse can last a lifetime if they're not treated properly.

Subtle forms of sexual abuse include inappropriate language, nudity, touching, or gazing. Mixed signals by caretakers that mask the perpetrator's sexual intent can be especially traumatic because the deception can disrupt trust. These activities can create confusion and insecurity in girls and young women at critical times in their emotional and mental development (Tjaden and Thoennes 1998).

What's important to remember when it comes to sexual trauma is that the wounds a survivor suffers are not directly proportional to the intensity of the physical act. Subtle abuse can have a more profound effect on a child, adolescent, or adult than overt sexual acts because of the long-term energetic problems created by the survivor's inability to connect the symptoms of sexual abuse to their cause.

To make matters worse, many adolescents and adults, because of embarrassment or fear of judgment and ostracism, choose to keep the abuse they experienced secret. However, no matter how a person rationalizes it, keeping the abuse secret will add a layer of shame. And shame will make it even more difficult for the survivor to overcome the effects of the original sexual trauma.

When shame has been added to the equation, there is only one remedy. A woman must personally confront the abuse by making contact with the woman she would've become if the abuse had never taken place. By doing that, the survivor can restore her authentic identity. Once her identity has been restored, the survivor will be able to manifest her soul urge and participate in intimate relationships without the legacy of the trauma getting in the way.

To overcome sexual trauma, you will release the intrusions first. Then you will decontaminate and reintegrate the energetic vehicles that were ejected. To restore the flow of prana through your energy field, you will activate your thirteen chakras and the first sex above body space. To overcome the legacy of shame caused by the sexual trauma, we've included the Personal Renewal Meditation. Perform the Personal Renewal Meditation after you've restored the flow of prana through your energy field.

---

## Exercise: The Personal Renewal Meditation

To perform the Personal Renewal Meditation, find a comfortable position with your back straight. Close your eyes and breathe deeply through your nose for two to three minutes. Then count backward from five to one and from ten to one. Use the Standard Method to relax your muscles and to center yourself in your authentic mind. Then assert, *"It's my intent to visualize a screen eight feet (two-and-a-half meters) in front of me."* Once the screen appears, assert, *"It's my intent to visualize the woman I would have become if I hadn't been sexually abused on the screen before me."* Immediately, an image of a woman will appear on the screen. She will be the woman you would've become if the abuse hadn't taken place. Observe her for a few moments. Pay attention to whether she can freely manifest all her functions of mind. Then ask yourself: Can the woman on the screen surrender more readily to intimacy than me? Does she appear more loving than me? Can she say "No" when it's appropriate? Does she manifest her authentic desires freely? Is she more self-reliant, flexible, and poised than I am now?

Once you've answered these questions, tell the woman on the screen what you experienced. Be specific. And don't leave out any details. Make sure you tell her how you felt during and after the abuse. When you're finished, choose a quality from your core field that has been blocked because of the abuse. It should be a quality you want to reassert more freely through your work and relationships.

The qualities that emerge through the core field include intent, will, desire, resistance, surrender, acceptance, knowing, choice, commitment, rejection, faith, enjoyment, destruction, empathy, creativity, and love.

Once you've chosen the quality you want to restore, assert, *"It's my intent to center myself in the section of my core field associated with (the quality you've chosen here)."* Once you're centered, continue by asserting, *"It's my intent to fill the section of my core field associated with (your choice here) with prana."* Don't do anything after that. Just enjoy the process for ten minutes. After ten minutes, assert, *"It's my intent to share the quality I've restored with the woman on my visual screen."* Take ten minutes to share the quality you've restored with the woman on the screen. After ten minutes, release the woman on the screen. Then release the screen. Take five minutes more to enjoy the shift you experience. Then count from one to five and bring yourself out of the meditation. Repeat as needed.

If you continue to practice the Personal Renewal Meditation until all your functions of mind have been restored, you will be able to manifest the universal qualities of the feminine without fear or shame disrupting your life and relationships.

## Summary

In this chapter, you learned how a traumatic experience can cripple a person on both the physical and subtle energetic levels. And, you learned to perform exercises designed to heal the energetic wounds that are common to all types of trauma. The exercises you learned enable you to release intrusions of distorted energy, heal fragmentation, and enhance the flow of prana through your energy field.

You also learned to heal the second-generation symptoms of trauma that emerge from the four most common traumatic events that people experience in the modern world.

In the next chapter, you will learn to enhance your fertility and to overcome the complications that accompany pregnancy, including cramps and panic attacks. You will also learn how to heal the energetic wounds caused by a miscarriage, abortion, or stillbirth.

# ELEVEN

# Healing Reproductive Wounds

In this chapter, we will examine fertility and the energetic wounds that can accompany pregnancy and birth. Then we will provide you with energetic solutions designed to enhance fertility and to heal those energetic wounds permanently. We will begin our examination by looking at fertility.

In the twenty-first century, fertility has become a major issue for women and couples who seek to have children and raise a family. In the United States alone, more than 10 percent of reproductive-age couples will have problems conceiving.

Many women who've had problems becoming pregnant have turned to fertility clinics. Although this is always an option, experience has taught us that the condition of a woman's energy field can have a significant effect on her ability to conceive and deliver a healthy baby.

To help women enhance their fertility, we've included an energetic regimen that we've used successfully with women who came to us for help. It has three parts. In the first part of the regimen, you will prepare and then consume fertility tea.

For those of you who've never used herbal teas for healing, it might surprise you to know that they have a long tradition in Asia, especially in Ayurvedic and Chinese medicine. They've been used to heal a host of conditions, promote good health, and enhance fertility.

## Fertility Tea

The preparation and the consumption of fertility tea are equally important. We recommend that you consider them both part of a sacred ritual. It's essential that you prepare the tea yourself without the interference of other people, your cell phone, computer, or television. To prepare fertility tea, you will need fifty grams of the following ingredients: Lady's Mantle (Alchemilla), St. John's Wort (Hypericum), Bedstraw (Galium), Herb Robert (Geranium robertianum), Yarrow (Achhilea millefolium), and Sweet Clover (Melilotus).

Once you've secured all the ingredients for your tea, mix them together so that they're ready to brew. One tablespoon will be enough to brew one large cup. Then use the Standard Method to relax your muscles and to center yourself in your authentic mind. Once you're centered, open your eyes and, for the next nine minutes, brew enough fertility tea for one large cup. When the tea is ready, drink it hot. Repeat the same process daily until you become pregnant (Trieb).

## Baby Wish Massage

Another technique that will enhance fertility is the baby wish massage. This is a massage that you will perform on yourself. The baby wish massage works because it increases as well as balances the flow of prana through a woman's reproductive organs, particularly her uterus. That in turn will enhance the health of her immune system and help reduce physical and psychological stress. It can also help to reposition a tilted uterus, improve poor circulation in the uterus and cervix, and promote a healthier hormonal balance.

---

### Exercise: Baby Wish Massage

We recommend that you use a natural oil with a pleasing scent for the baby wish massage and that you practice it two or three times a week until you become pregnant. We also recommend that you drink a cup of fertility tea after you've completed your massage.

Heat up the room you will use for the massage before you begin. Then lie down on your back. Use the Standard Method to relax your muscles and center yourself in your authentic mind. Then liberally apply the oil on the skin above your abdomen and pelvis. With the palm of your positive hand, right hand if you're right-handed, left hand if you're left-handed, begin to massage your pelvis. After a couple of minutes, move your hand diagonally along your hip bones, first on the right side and then on the left side of your pelvis. Repeat three times. Then cup your positive hand and, using it like a shovel, pull it upward from the mount of Venus to your solar plexus. Apply enough pressure so that you can feel the muscles of your uterus relaxing. As your confidence grows, you can apply more pressure with the side of your hand. Inhale on each stroke while you let your breath lead you upward.

We've found that twenty strokes are usually sufficient to relax the uterus. After you've made twenty strokes upward, bring both hands to the mount of Venus. Then slowly separate them and move them across your abdomen toward the high points on your hip bones. While you move them, use your index, middle, and ring fingers of each hand to make small circular movements.

By using your fingertips like a laser pointer, you will feel concentrations of distorted energy and karmic baggage buried in the deep tissues. Next, use your intent and mental attention to surround each concentration of distorted energy with a prana box. Then perform the Orgasmic Bliss Mudra (go to chapter 4). And while you hold it, assert, *"It's my intent to fill all the prana boxes I created with bliss and to release all the distorted energy within them."* After you're finished, close your eyes and take ten minutes to enjoy the changes you experience. Then count from one to five and bring yourself out of the exercise. After the massage, have a cup of fertility tea.

## Exercise to Enhance Fertility

The exercise to enhance fertility will enhance the flow of feminine energy through your reproductive organs. That in turn will enhance the processes of fertilization and conception. The exercise has three parts.

In the first part, you will use your intent and mental attention to create a visual screen. Then you will use your intent and mental attention to create an energetic brush to clean out your ovaries, fallopian tubes, and uterus. In the second part, you will fill your ovaries with prana. In the third part you will activate your second and fifth chakras and center yourself in the corresponding chakra fields.

To begin the exercise, find a comfortable position with your back straight. Close your eyes and breathe deeply through your nose for two to three minutes. Then count backward from five to one and from ten to one. Use the Standard Method to relax your muscles and to center yourself in your authentic mind. Then assert, *"It's my intent to create a visual screen eight feet (two-and-a-half meters) in front of me."* Continue by asserting, *"It's my intent to visualize an image of myself on the screen in front of me."* Next, assert, *"It's my intent to create an energetic brush."* As soon as the energetic brush appears, take hold of it and use it to brush your ovaries, fallopian tubes, and uterus clean. After you're satisfied that your reproductive organs have been cleansed of all impurities, release your cleansing tool and assert, *"It's my intent to fill my reproductive organs with prana."* Continue to fill them with prana until they begin to glow with energy. Then assert, *"It's my intent to activate my second chakra."* Next, assert, *"It's my intent to center myself in my second chakra field."* Once you're centered in your second chakra field, assert, *"It's my intent to activate my fifth chakra."* Then assert, *"It's my intent to center myself in my fifth chakra field."* Take ten minutes to enjoy the enhanced glow of energy you feel in your chakras and reproductive organs. After ten minutes, release the image of yourself on the screen and the visual screen. Then count from one to five and bring yourself out of the meditation. Repeat every day until you become pregnant.

## Pregnancy

Pregnancy can be a challenge for any women. It makes demands on a woman's body and energy field. And it divides her attention, making it even harder for her to devote herself to her career and care for her family. Adding to a woman's burden during pregnancy are abdominal cramps and panic attacks. Since these conditions have an energetic foundation and afflict so many pregnant women, we've included exercises designed specifically to overcome them.

## Cramps During Pregnancy

Abdominal cramps during pregnancy can be so painful that they can disable a woman. In order to overcome abdominal cramps, we've developed the Abdominal Relief Mudra. The Abdominal Relief Mudra will enhance the flow of prana through your pelvis and promote the flow of energy through the chakras that supply your abdomen with prana, including the second chakra, the lower etheric chakra, the lower physical chakra, and the lower physical material chakra. The mudra also stimulates the acupuncture point in the colon, which releases prana from the first chakra and stimulates the kundalini-shakti, one of the most powerful forms of feminine energy in your energy field.

You can use the mudra to relieve pain as soon as you feel the onset of cramps. In that case, hold the mudra for at least ten minutes and repeat every half hour until the cramps no longer disturb you. If you practice the mudra regularly (once a day) when you become pregnant, it's possible to avoid cramps altogether.

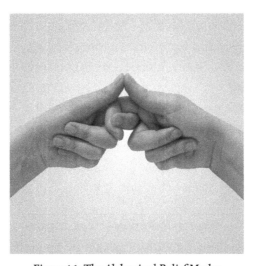

*Figure 16: The Abdominal Relief Mudra*

---

### Exercise: Abdominal Relief Mudra

To begin the Abdominal Relief Mudra, find a comfortable position with your back straight. Then close your eyes and breathe deeply through your nose for two to three minutes. Use the Standard Method to relax your muscles and to center yourself in your authentic mind. Then place the tips of your index fingers together. Continue by placing the tips of your thumbs together.

Bend the middle fingers, ring fingers and pinky of each hand into the palms and apply a little pressure to the mount of Venus (the base of your thumb) with your curled fingertips. Hold the mudra for at ten minutes and repeat every day while you're pregnant.

## Panic Attacks During Pregnancy

Panic attacks are essentially episodes of intense mental stress combined with physical symptoms that can be so overwhelming, they overload a woman's nervous system.

Why people have panic attacks remains a mystery to scientists and medical practitioners. However, from our research we've learned that because of hormonal fluctuations during pregnancy, energetic traumas, the reemergence of karmic issues, and the energetic wounds that support them, the flow of prana can become blocked. Add to that the increased sensitivity and fear a woman can have when she's pregnant as well as the loss of freedom, it's not surprising that some women experience panic attacks.

To overcome panic attacks, we've developed the Panic Attack Mudra. It's designed specifically to prevent a woman's energy field from becoming overloaded. Once you've learned to perform the mudra, you will combine it with two other activities, which you can use when a panic attack is imminent or has already begun.

---

### Exercise: Panic Attack Mudra

To perform the Panic Attack Mudra, find a comfortable position with your back straight. Keep the soles of your feet on the floor and your tongue in its normal position. Then close your eyes and breathe deeply through your nose for two to three minutes. Use the Standard Method to relax your muscles and to center yourself in your authentic mind. Then bring the tip of your tongue to the top of your mouth. Next slide it back until the palate becomes soft and hold it there. Then cross your right thumb over your left thumb. Next, bend your index fingers and press them together from the tip to the first joint. Then create two triangles by placing the tips of your middle fingers together and by placing the tips of your ring fingers together. Bend your pinkies and bring them together so that they're touching from the first to the second joint. Hold the mudra from ten minutes. Repeat as needed.

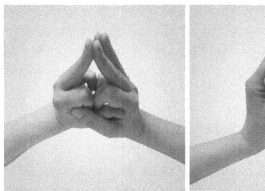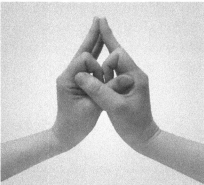

*Figure 17: The Panic Attack Mudra*

## Emergency Treatment for a Panic Attack

When a panic attack is imminent or has already begun, we recommend that you do three things. First take a shower with cold water. This will saturate your body with negative ions. Negative ions will increase the level of the mood-enhancing chemical serotonin in your brain. That will help to relieve stress and boost energy; both will help you overcome panic attacks.

After you've showered for a few minutes, sit down in a comfortable place and perform the Panic Attack Mudra. Hold the mudra while you activate your third chakra. Then center yourself in your third chakra field. Once you're centered in your third chakra field, release the mudra and begin to chant ohm from your third chakra until calm has been restored.

Ohm is the cosmic sound. It emerged when the universe was created. Its therapeutic effect is well known especially when it's used with the appropriate meditations and mudras.

## Miscarriage, Abortion, and Stillbirth

For women, especially those experiencing their first pregnancy, losing a baby by miscarriage, stillbirth, or abortion can be an especially traumatic event. In the following pages, we will do our best to explain what happens when a child is lost, by looking into what happens energetically to a woman and her unborn child. Then we will provide you with exercises to heal the wounds of miscarriage, stillbirth and abortion. This will enable you to release the painful legacy of these events. And it will help the soul of your unborn child proceed joyfully on its evolutionary journey.

## The Energetic Legacy of Miscarriage, Abortion, and Stillbirth

Although some women may suffer physically for years after the loss of a child, it's not the physical costs alone that pose a threat to women. The psychological and energetic effects can be devastating as well for the woman, her unborn child, and her family (Pro Femina).

For many women, the process of grieving begins immediately after the loss of the child as a reflex to the physical, psychological, and energetic trauma. A woman may try to repress or control the sadness and grief that is inevitable, but it normally doesn't work very well. That's because the energetic wounds underlying the loss are rarely healed. As a result, many women suffer from unresolved feelings of self-recrimination and longing, and respond by isolating themselves afterward from friends and family.

From an energetic perspective, the loss of a child through miscarriage, abortion, or stillbirth is a severe trauma for both mother and child. That's because a mother's dharma and her purpose for incarnating are closely linked to the karmic connection she has to her unborn child. When a child is lost, the connection they have to one another is broken. And that has far-reaching consequences for both the unborn child and its mother.

## Tamara's Story

Tamara's experience illustrates how traumatic the loss of an unborn child can be. We began working with Tamara in 2010, when she was thirty-four.

After working with us almost a year, she visited a fertility clinic and with its help she become pregnant. Six months into the pregnancy, her water broke while she was at the airport. She was treated almost immediately, but she lost her son in the ambulance on the way to the hospital.

The loss of her son had a profound effect on her. Almost immediately she shut down and withdrew from her family and friends. She remained chronically depressed for several months and her hormone levels remained so unbalanced that she continued to produce milk for almost a year.

After several months, she began to open up and we began to treat her for the energetic trauma she and her unborn son had experienced. To bring her hormones back in balance, we treated her with Hormeel, an alternative homeopathic medicine. Then we provided her with a regimen of energy work, which she practiced for twelve weeks. During that time, she restored her life-affirming identity by removing intrusions and reintegrating three energetic vehicles. She successfully activated her second and fifth chakras and centered herself in their corresponding energy fields. She created a prana bandage (see page 155) to heal the wound in her pelvis. And she used the techniques we taught her to let go of the son and help his soul proceed joyfully on its journey.

Five months into the work, she told us that she was pregnant. We discontinued our work at that point. Eight months later, we learned that she'd delivered a healthy baby boy.

## The Energetic Cost to the Mother

Although people continue to debate when the soul of the unborn arrives in the womb, our work with women indicates that an energetic link is established very early in the pregnancy.

As soon as this link is established, a transfer begins and elements of the child's soul, including energetic vehicles, start to descend into the developing fetus. If the process is interrupted by a miscarriage or abortion, and in some cases a stillbirth, some energetic vehicles will remain stuck in the mother's energy field, some will be lost in transit, and others will remain in the unborn waiting vainly to descend.

The energy bodies that have already descended into the mother's body cannot easily reunite with the unborn after a miscarriage, abortion, or stillbirth has occurred. In most cases, they will get stuck within the mother's energy field, which explains why most women who've had a miscarriage, abortion, or stillbirth carry an attachment to the unborn for years afterward.

The energy bodies stuck in transit will also be affected. They will be cut off from the resource fields that normally provide them with energy and consciousness. These bodies will frantically look for a safe haven, one that will provide them with the energy and consciousness they need. Some of these energy bodies will find a dubious safety in other people's energy fields. Other energy bodies will be violated by predatory fields of energy and consciousness that feed on the prana they contain. Energy bodies that remain in the mother or find safety in other people will create unhealthy attachments between the unborn and its host or hosts.

These attachments can last for lifetimes because each energy body is connected to the energy field of the soul by a silver cord. Silver cords are an essential part of the unborn's non-physical anatomy. Eventually, when the soul of the unborn child finds another mother in which to incarnate, it will feel the loss of these bodies and will do its best to find them and reintegrate them. But without the knowledge and skill to do so, its task will be difficult to accomplish.

In order to heal the wounds to both mother and child, we've included a series of exercises designed specifically to help them both overcome the trauma caused by a miscarriage, abortion, or stillbirth.

The series includes an exercise to release your attachment to the soul of the unborn as well as a prana bandage to heal the energetic wound suffered by the mother. It also includes an exercise to help the unborn child complete its life journey with all its energy bodies intact.

## Exercise: Releasing the Soul of the Unborn

You should release your attachment to the soul of your unborn if she or he was lost due to negligence on your part or because you had an abortion. If you feel guilty for the loss of a child you should also release your attachment to the soul of your unborn. Releasing the attachment to your unborn child accomplishes several things that are karmically important. If the mother was responsible, it acknowledges that fact and it offers sincere regrets for the disruption of the child's life journey. If the mother wasn't at fault, it allows her to let go of the guilt and shame she carries, so that she can complete the process of self-healing.

To be effective the process must remove both the karmic attachment and erase the karmic debt. And it must be given freely. The process has two parts. In the first part you must accurately describe the actions that violated the unborn child. In the second part must express the sincere regret you feel for harming the unborn child energetically and for preventing the child from incarnating on earth.

When you're ready to begin, sit down in a quiet place. Then close your eyes and breathe deeply through your nose for two to three minutes. Count backward from five to one and from ten to one. Then use the Standard Method to relax your muscles and to center yourself in your authentic mind.

Once you're relaxed, assert, *"It's my intent to activate my heart chakra."* Then assert, *"It's my intent to center myself in my heart chakra field."* Continue by asserting, *"It's my intent to turn my organs of perception inward on the level of my heart chakra."* Take a moment to enjoy the shift. Then assert,

*"It's my intent to visualize a screen eight feet (two-and-a-half meters) in front of me."* Continue by asserting, *"It's my intent to visualize my unborn child on the screen in front of me."* The child will appear on the screen at the appropriate age to continue its journey.

To release the attachment assert, *"I'm sincerely sorry for causing you pain and for playing a part in disrupting your life's journey."* Look directly at the child when you make your assertion. Once you're done and you can sense that the child has accepted your sincere regrets, you can say good-bye to your unborn. To do that, you will radiate energy from your heart chakra to the child. And when your unborn child accepts it, assert, *"I set you free to continue your evolutionary journey, good-bye."* Then release the child, and release the screen. Bring yourself out of the meditation by counting from one to five.

After the unborn has accepted your regrets, you can help it proceed joyfully on its life journey by returning energetic vehicles from your unborn that remain trapped in your energy field.

---

### Exercise: Helping the Child
### Complete its Life Journey

To begin the process, fill a hot bath with Dead Sea salt (you can buy Dead Sea salt in any health food store or pharmacy). Then lie in the bath with your legs spread apart. Close your eyes and breathe deeply through your nose for two to three minutes. Then count backward from five to one and from ten to one. Use the Standard Method to relax your muscles and to center yourself in your authentic mind.

Then assert, *"It's my intent that the salt in my bath absorbs all the distorted energy associated with the loss of my unborn child."* Sea salt has the ability to absorb distorted energy on the physical material, physical, and etheric levels. Take five minutes to enjoy the process. Then assert, *"It's my intent surround all the energetic vehicles of my unborn child in my energy field with prana boxes."* Then perform the Orgasmic Bliss Mudra (go to chapter 4). Hold the mudra while you assert, *"It's my intent that bliss decontaminates all the energetic vehicles of my unborn in my energy field and that all the energetic vehicles that remain within it return directly to their appropriate place in the universe."* Release the mudra next. Then lie in the water for fifteen minutes and allow the energetic vehicles of your unborn to be cleansed and to reunite with its soul. Repeat until you know that the unborn child is once more proceeding joyfully on its life journey. You will know that that process is complete when you no longer feel an unhealthy attachment to your unborn.

## Exercise: The Prana Bandage

The final exercise in this chapter is a prana bandage. A prana bandage will have a profound impact on your psychological health and the health of your energy field because it will seal the energetic wound created by a miscarriage, stillbirth, or abortion. Creating a prana bandage is a five-day process.

### Day 1

To begin the process on day one, find a comfortable position with your back straight. Close your eyes and breathe deeply through your nose for two to three minutes. Then count backward from five to one and from ten to one. Use the Standard Method to relax your muscles and to center yourself in your authentic mind. Then assert, *"It's my intent to visualize a screen eight feet (two-and-a-half meters) in front of me."* Continue by asserting, *"It's my intent to visualize myself on the screen."* Once you appear on the screen, assert, *"It's my intent to visualize that my abdomen is surrounded by a bandage made of prana."* After you've created the bandage, take ten minutes more to enjoy the process. After ten minutes, release the image of yourself and the screen. Then bring yourself out of the meditation by counting from one to five.

### Days 2–4

On days two, three, and four, find a comfortable position with your back straight. Close your eyes and breathe deeply through your nose for two to three minutes. Then count backward from five to one and from ten to one. Use the Standard Method to relax your muscles and to center yourself in your authentic mind. Then assert, *"It's my intent to visualize a screen eight feet (two-and-a-half meters) in front of me."* Continue by asserting, *"It's my intent to visualize myself on the screen."* Then assert, *"It's my intent to replace my old prana bandage with a new one."* After you've replaced the prana bandage with a new one, assert, *"It's my intent to fill my uterus and vagina with prana."* Take ten minutes more to enjoy the process. After ten minutes, release the image of yourself and the screen. Then bring yourself out of the meditation by counting from one to five.

### Day 5

On day five, find a comfortable position with your back straight. Close your eyes and breathe deeply through your nose for two to three minutes. Then count backward from five to one and from ten to one. Use the Standard Method to relax your muscles and to center yourself in your authentic mind. Then assert, *"It's my intent to visualize a screen eight feet (two-and-a-half meters) in front of me."* Continue by asserting, *"It's my intent to visualize myself on the screen."* Once you appear on the screen, assert, *"It's my intent to replace my old prana bandage with a new one."* After you've replaced the prana bandage with a new one, assert, *"It's my intent to fill my uterus and vagina with prana."* After that, visualize that the prana that has filled your uterus and vagina has radiated into your prana bandage and created one large field of prana that fills your abdomen.

Take ten minutes more to enjoy the process. Then release both the image of yourself and the visual screen. To complete the process, count from one to five. Then open your eyes and bring yourself out of the meditation. Repeat as needed.

## Summary

In this chapter, you learned to use simple remedies and exercises to enhance your fertility. Then you learned to heal the complications that can accompany pregnancy, including cramps and panic attacks.

Finally, you learned how to heal the wounds created by the loss of an unborn child. In the next chapter, you will learn to recover your sexual power by making room for passion. Then you will learn to enhance the flow of prana through your sexual organs. Finally, you will learn to enhance your sexual desire so that you can experience more joy and intimacy in your relationships.

# TWELVE

## Restoring Your Sexual Power

Helen F. Fisher wrote in *The Sex Contract: The Evolution of Human Behavior,*

> Our species is consecrated to sex, we speak and laugh about it, we sing about it, we make love regularly ... Why? Because a woman can maintain a permanent state of arousal. Physically she can make love every day of her adult life, even when she is pregnant.

While no other species has a female that is genetically programmed for love and eroticism, it's rare to see a woman who is satisfied with her sexual life. There are two reasons for that. The first is that most women have had their natural eroticism and sensuality blocked by disruptions in their energy field. The second is that many institutions in society still don't honor a woman's natural power, creativity, and radiance.

Although many women in modern technological societies believe that they are sexually liberated, the uncomfortable truth is that, in most parts of the world, the core values of society still support a social contract that sees women as either weak and dependent, or as sexual objects.

Since there is so little support for the healthy expression of a woman's natural eroticism and sensuality, modern women have few choices. Many women play the world's game and substitute lust and control for eroticism and sensuality. Unfortunately, as a relationship strategy, that won't work for very long because eroticism and sensuality are hard-wired into a woman's physical body and energy field. And the substitution of lust and control won't satisfy a woman on the deeper levels of soul and spirit.

In her informative book *The Woman's Encyclopedia of Myths and Secrets*, Barbara G. Walker calls eroticism in today's world "the final pursuit of shock, destruction, and death." She adds that

> Any woman paying attention will recognize that in Western society the male aspects of eroticism and sensuality are over emphasized, making sexuality overly permissive, degrading and pornographic. This can be seen in how sexuality is expressed in the media, pornography, in books and movies, the Internet—and how the idea that lust and libertine sexual activities divorced from intimacy constitute sexual liberation. (Walker 2007, 1019–1020)

No serious woman could possibly believe that. Ask yourself: Is a woman sexually liberated when she still doesn't listen to her authentic needs or to what nourishes and satisfies her? Or has she merely become a stereotype of a society, still interested in portraying women as sexy and lustful, indulging in all kinds of sexual behavior even if it doesn't satisfy her deepest needs for love and intimacy?

The truth is that neither the suppression of female desire nor the acceptance of a male view of sensuality and eroticism can be an appropriate model for a radiant woman. The radiant woman is someone who uses her natural sensuality and eroticism to dive into the current of life, where the spirits of men and women come into union and are carried away in rapture.

## Katerina's Story

The story of Katerina illustrates how a woman's life and relationships can be disrupted by sexist values. Katerina was thirty-three years old when she came to us for help. Her early childhood was scarred by a father who sexually abused her. Like many women, she was so ashamed by what took place that she kept the abuse secret.

Because of the karmic wound she'd suffered and the lack of trust in herself and in men, her sexuality became a simple commodity that she sold to the highest bidder. She used her rage, which she had in abundance, to good effect, too. It became the foundation of a lustful persona that would appeal to powerful older men who she intuitively knew would serve as her sugar daddy. Sex was the currency she used to hold on to men and get what she wanted from them.

She continued this pattern until she got pregnant. When she demanded that the child's father support her, he refused. And when she forced the issue by refusing to sleep with him, he responded by leaving her.

Eventually, she met another man who challenged her emotionally. Insecurity and fear emerged almost immediately and became so intense that she finally broke down and came to us for help.

It wasn't until her fourth session that she told us about the sexual abuse. At the end of the session we taught her two exercises designed to heal the energetic wounds she'd suffered and to overcome the sexist view of female sexuality that had dominated her life for so long. Since then she has made remarkable progress, and has been able to participate in an intimate relationship with her new partner. The relationship still has challenges, but it has become healthier as Katerina successfully works through her relationship issues. Katerina now raises her daughter in Berlin with partner Sebastian.

## Making Room for Passion

In a society where institutions still support sexist values, lust is highly valued by many people. It replaces authentic passion and pleasure, love, intimacy, and joy, which are its true companions and which nourish a woman's soul and spirit. If lust dominates a woman, then intimacy will be squeezed out of her intimate relationships and the satisfaction that comes from intimacy and authentic passion will evaporate along with her sensitivity to her own body.

To help you overcome the distorted energy that supports lust and heal your soul from its legacy, we've included the Freedom from Lust

Meditation. The Freedom from Lust Meditation will help you enhance the functions of your light body field so that you can replace lust with authentic passion.

The light body field is a resource field with a vibration one step higher than the core field. Like the core field, it fills your energy field and physical body, and extends beyond it in all directions.

By enhancing the functions of the light body field and centering yourself in it, you will find a place within your soul where lust is superseded by authentic passion and your authentic feminine qualities emerge without distortion.

---

### Exercise: The Freedom from Lust Meditation

To begin the Freedom from Lust Meditation, sit in a comfortable position with your back straight. Close your eyes and breathe deeply through your nose for two to three minutes. Then count backward from five to one and from ten to one. Use the Standard Method to relax your muscles and to center yourself in your authentic mind. Then assert, *"It's my intent to center myself in my light body field."* Continue by asserting, *"It's my intent to fill my light body field with prana."* After you've filled the light body field with prana, assert, *"It's my intent to turn my organs of perception inward on the level of my light body field."* Take ten minutes to enjoy the process. Then count from one to five and bring yourself out of the meditation. Repeat the meditation every day until lust no longer disrupts you, or interferes with your natural sexual passion.

### A Life of Passion

Women weren't always trapped by the same distorted sexual patterns that trapped Katerina. In the Orient, in early historical times, there was a very different view of female eroticism and sensuality. For the ancestral woman, sex wasn't about lust and chasing orgasms. Instead, it was a slowly unfolding series of activities—mental, emotional, sensual, and sexual—that allowed her to intimately experience her partner and share her sexual passion with him (Walker 2007, 1019–1020.)

Partners approached each other with their senses open and active, and shared prana freely. Their intimate dance allowed them to surrender to the profound pleasure and relaxation that brought them into balance and healed them on all levels.

Çatal Höyük, the Mediterranean city in Anatolia, is thought to have been a city where partners openly expressed their sensuality and explored their sexual relationships with passion and freedom. It has been described as a Tantric city because researchers have found that the city was filled with relics that honored fertility and the Mother Goddess (Lysebeth 1990).

The fall of Çatal Höyük is still a mystery. But what we do know is that, in many modern societies, sexuality and a women's role in it have become objectified. As a result, couples will try almost anything to feel satisfied and achieve intimacy, from bondage, dildos, and submissive-dominance games to adult movies.

Unfortunately, despite all these sexual tools and techniques, rarely are women or men satisfied with their sexual lives. This leads to relationships where intimacy and authentic sharing is the exception rather than the rule.

The time has come to recognize that a sexual life that remains unbalanced can never satisfy a woman who seeks to become radiant. That's because a radiant woman experiences her body and her sexuality differently. Her eroticism is not based on lust and control but on intimacy and the wellspring of feminine energy that grants sexual power and passion.

Now that you've performed the Freedom from Lust Meditation, you're ready to recover your sexual power and passion by practicing the regimen of exercises we've included in the following pages. In the first exercise, the Yoni Mudra, you will take back control of the pleasure centers in your body and energy field.

---

## Exercise: The Yoni Mudra

*Yoni* is a Sanskrit word that means "divine passage" or "place of birth." On the physical level, it corresponds to a woman's vagina. In a wider context, it also means origin, fountain, or sacred space: the space occupied by a radiant woman in her fullness, both as the manifestation of the universal feminine and as the wellspring of sexual pleasure. Women who practice the Yoni Mudra will experience the benefits that come from experiencing and expressing pleasure fully.

To perform the Yoni Mudra, find a comfortable position with your back straight. Then close your eyes and breathe deeply through your nose for two to three minutes. Use the Standard Method to relax your muscles and to center yourself in your authentic mind. Then bring your hands together, palms open and facing each other at a slight angle. Interlock your pinkies together at the first joint. Then cross your ring fingers behind your middle fingers. Your middle finger should be fully extended and touching at the tips. Your ring fingers will be held down by the index fingers. Your thumbs will be curled into the palms.

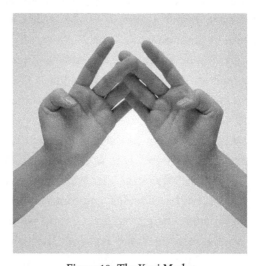

*Figure 18: The Yoni Mudra*

If you perform the Yoni Mudra for ten minutes a day for two weeks, you will experience more pleasure and have more freedom to express your natural eroticism and sexual passion. Repeat as needed.

Taking back control of the pleasure centers is a prerequisite for a healthy and joyful sexuality in which your natural eroticism and sexual passion are given free reign to radiate. Once you've liberated the pleasure centers in your energy field and physical body, you're ready to enhance your sexual desire.

## Enhancing Sexual Desire

Unfortunately, many women assume it's natural to lose sexual desire after childbirth because of familiarity, or during and after menopause. However, the loss of sexual desire need not accompany any of these phases in a woman's life. Sexual desire is related more to the condition of a woman's energy field than any physical events, even those related to the production of hormones in a woman's body.

Medical research has shown that the production of hormones, even those related to sexual pleasure, is affected by a woman's mental state (and therefore her energetic condition). Dr. Doris Wolf, a psychologist at the University of Heidelberg, states, "The production of sexual hormones, which leads to sexual pleasure, is inspired by thought and fantasy. The movie of the mind is the Viagra of body—the fuel that makes the hormones do their dance."

Since psychological and subtle energetic factors play an important part in women's libido, sexual desire is not necessarily diminished as a woman gets older. While it's true that sexual desire in women awakens a bit later than in men, women need not experience a decline in sexual desire during or after menopause when the estrogen levels decline and the ovaries produce less testosterone. The fact is that mature women have more time to focus on themselves and their sex life. As a result, a woman's love life and her sexual desire can blossom during any stage of her life, even during and after menopause.

Since it's energy with universal qualities that supports a woman's sexual desire and a woman's natural eroticism, by enhancing that energy in the appropriate way, a woman's natural eroticism and sexuality can be enhanced.

To do that, you will perform the same two exercises that helped Katerina and Sebastian enhance their authentic sexual desire for each other.

The first exercise is called the Yoni Meditation. The Yoni Meditation will help increase sexual desire before and during sex. And it will enhance the satisfaction you feel when a man enters you and shares his sexual energy with you.

---

## Exercise: The Yoni Meditation

To perform the Yoni Meditation, sit or lie in a comfortable position with your back straight. Close your eyes and breathe deeply through your nose for two to three minutes. Then count backward from five to one and from ten to one. Use the Standard Method to relax your muscles and to center yourself in your authentic mind. Then bring your mental attention to your vagina. Next, assert, *"It's my intent that, on each inhalation, prana flows directly to my vagina and the energy centers that support it."* Once you feel your vagina vibrating or glowing with prana, squeeze the muscles in your vagina together. Mentally count from one to seven while you increase the pressure in your vagina. Then exhale through your mouth and relax the muscles of your vagina for a count of seven. Repeat twenty-five times. Then breathe normally and let your muscles relax for another ten minutes while you enjoy the enhanced prana and sexual desire that radiates through your vagina and the energy centers in your pelvis. After ten minutes, count from one to five. Then open your eyes and bring yourself out of the meditation. Repeat as needed.

Once you've increased your own sexual desire, you can do the same for your partner because your networks and sheaths connect you together.

---

## Exercise: Increasing Your Partner's Sexual Desire

Before you attempt to increase your partner's sexual desire, get his permission. Then instruct him to close his eyes and breathe deeply through the nose for the duration of the exercise.

Once your partner is relaxed, close your eyes and breathe deeply through your nose for two to three minutes. Then count backward from five to one and from ten to one. Use the Standard Method to relax your muscles and to center yourself in your authentic mind. Then assert, *"It's my intent to activate my second chakra."* Take a few moments to enjoy the shift. Then assert, *"It's my intent to center myself in my second chakra field."* Once you're centered in your second chakra field, bring your attention to your vagina. Breathe into your vagina so that prana fills it on each inhalation. Once you feel your vagina vibrating or glowing with prana, pull the energy from your vagina up to your eyes on each exhalation.

When you feel sexual energy and desire emerging through your eyes, open them and gaze at your partner. Continue gazing for ten minutes, or as long as you feel comfortable. Then count from one to five and bring yourself out of the meditation. To bring your partner out of the meditation, have him count from one to five and open his eyes.

You can use the partner variation of the Yoni Meditation as part of your regimen of energy work or before you engage in sex. In either case, if your partner is open and receptive, you will quickly enhance his desire, and both of you will experience a much more satisfying sexual relationship.

## Conflicting Desires and Sexual Performance

Sexual desire is a complex issue for many women. Like Katerina, many women continue to have their natural desires suppressed or distorted by karmic energy and restrictive beliefs. Distorted desires can easily come into conflict with a woman's natural passion and desire for sexual intimacy. They can also interfere with a woman's ability to manifest her radiance. After all, a woman with a conflicted mind cannot manifest or share her passion freely.

In order for a woman to recover her natural sexual passion, she must overcome the conflicting desires that emerge from karmic baggage and restrictive beliefs. This is true even for liberated woman living in the twenty-first century. That's because all women have lived before and, as a result, all women have been influenced by the cultural and religious conditioning they experienced in the past.

## Sexual Desire and Breasts

Contrary to what most people believe, the primary source of a woman's sexual desire and passion is not a woman's clitoris, but her breasts.

Women are sexually aroused more quickly and thoroughly when their breasts are stimulated than any other part of their body.

There are several reasons for this. A woman's breasts correspond to her heart chakra. The heart chakra, as you recall, regulates a woman's rights, which include the right to be herself and the right to express herself as the erotic, sensual woman she was born to be. There is also a polar relationship between a woman's breasts and her vagina. A woman is masculine and asserts prana and her natural feminine power through her breasts. And she is feminine and accepts prana through her vagina. This means that a woman's ability to assert her natural feminine power is more closely associated with her breasts than her vagina.

Men recognize this on an unconscious level, which explains why men are so interested in a woman's breasts, as both sexual objects and objects of nourishment. Breasts also interest men because they're not only the outer manifestation of the heart chakra; they're the outer manifestation of the human heart, on the left side of the heart chakra, and the divine heart, Atman, on the right side. This means that a woman's breasts are associated with love because of their relationship to the human heart, with intimacy because of their relationship to the heart chakra, and with transcendence because of their relationship to Atman.

Most men, because of their conditioning, may not express their yearning for these three things. But as every woman knows, when stripped to the core most men yearn for them.

Unfortunately, many women have had their relationship to their breasts disrupted. That's because modern Western societies objectify breasts, separating them from the women who possess them. This makes them objects of lust, which can disrupt a woman's relationship to them. When a woman's relationship to her breasts has been disturbed, a woman's relationship to her three hearts (her human heart, heart chakra, and Atman) will be disrupted and so will her ability to assert her personal rights, including her right to express her sexual passion freely.

## Loving Your Breasts Again

Regardless of the conflicted relationship modern Western societies have with breasts, you can use them, and the energy radiating through them, to restore your natural sexual desire.

In the following exercise you will learn to love them again so that you can radiate prana from your three hearts freely, without distortion. This in turn will enhance your sexual desire and passion.

You may not realize it, but you continually love the body parts that give you pleasure by allowing prana to radiate through them. The energy that radiates through those body parts provides them with the nourishment they need to function healthfully and maintain a healthy relationship to the rest of your energy field and physical body. When prana radiates freely through your breasts, you will enjoy how they feel, how they look, and your natural sexual desire will emerge through them without disruption.

In contrast, cultural conditioning, karmic baggage, and the after-effects of trauma can all interfere with a woman's relationship to her breasts. They can make a woman disapprove, neglect, or deny love to her breasts, or make a woman believe that her breasts are unattractive.

Regardless of the reasons why you disapprove, neglect, or deny love to your breasts, by doing so, you will restrict the flow of prana radiating through them, and that will force the energy emerging through your breasts to contract. Once it has contracted, your breasts will respond either by becoming overly sensitive or by losing sensation and becoming numb.

---

## Exercise: Breast Meditation

In the Breast Meditation, you will fill your breasts with prana. Once you've filled your breasts with prana, they will radiate freely on their own, and they will automatically integrate their energy with the energy radiating through your other body parts so that you can share your natural sexual desire freely.

To begin the exercise, find a comfortable position with your back straight. Close your eyes and breathe deeply through your nose for two to three minutes. Then count backward from five to one and from ten to one. Use the Standard Method to relax your muscles and to center yourself in your authentic mind. Then assert, *"It's my intent to activate my heart chakra."* Continue by asserting, *"It's my intent to center myself in my heart chakra field."* Take a few moments to enjoy the shift. Then assert, *"It's my intent to focus my mental attention on my breasts and fill them with prana."* Once you've asserted your intent, relax. Prana will fill your breasts without any further effort on your part.

Allow the process to continue for ten minutes while your mental attention remains focused on your breasts. After ten minutes, count from one to five. When you reach the number five, open your eyes. You will feel wide-awake, perfectly relaxed, and better than you did before.

You may have to repeat the exercise several times before your breasts radiate prana freely. However, if you practice the exercise regularly, it won't be long before your sexual desire emerges naturally and you can freely share it with your partner.

## Summary

In this chapter, you recovered your authentic sexual passion by performing the Freedom from Lust Meditation, the Yoni Mudra, and by enhancing the flow of prana through your sexual organs. You also learned to enhance your sexual desire and your partner's sexual desire so that you can share more intimacy and love in your sexual relationship.

In the following chapter, you will learn how to enhance your healing power. You will do that by creating your own healing space and by learning to heal yourself and those you love on the levels of body, mind, and spirit.

After that, you will learn how to liberate the power within the menstrual blood. To facilitate that process, we've developed an exercise called the Cycle of Life Meditation. It will help you to overcome negative feelings and thoughts associated with menstruation and to recognize that the menstrual cycle is a manifestation of a woman's power, creativity, and radiance.

## THIRTEEN

# Enhancing Your
# Healing Power

Women in matriarchal societies were secure in the knowledge that they were natural healers. That's because the prana they used for healing came directly from the universal feminine. Unfortunately, in the modern world most women have difficulty manifesting their healing power for the same reasons they have trouble manifesting their creativity. For centuries, the power of women to heal and to create has been a threat to societies that did not honor a woman's natural strengths and abilities.

In the West, the demonization of women who used their power to heal is a long, tragic story. It began with the destruction of matriarchal societies. But it gathered steam in the Middle Ages when healers and midwives were systematically persecuted.

Although any woman who healed could become a target in the Middle Ages, many women in esoteric circles and in secret societies across Europe and the Middle East continued to heal. But rarely did they recognize that turning to spirits and energetic fields outside their own healing space prevented them from reaching their potential as healers and as women. The situation continued with little change until the nineteenth century when a remarkable shift in medical science took place. The shift was caused by the introduction of the germ theory. The germ theory was the brainchild of Louis Pasteur, who taught that it was the presence of microbes in the human body that caused disease.

Once this new paradigm took root, the practice of medicine became more mechanical—and more divorced from a woman's healing space. Since then, the importance of a woman's healing space has almost been completely overlooked. And the subtle energy that women use to heal took a back seat to the novel concept that there was a simple cause and effect relationship between microbes in the human body and health. Wellness, diet, and lifestyle were ignored almost entirely as factors until the end of the twentieth century.

Even today, when the presence of healing energy is the only rational explanation for the placebo effect, and medical practitioners know that for every human cell there are ten times the number of helpful microbes living in the human body, many people still believe that a drug prescription will solve all their ills.

To illustrate how important a woman's healing space can be we've included Sabrina's story.

## Sabrina's Story

In our first meeting Sabrina told us that when she was six years old she had an infected tooth, which was extremely painful. Instead of crying and running to her mother for help she quietly went to her room. Then she sat down and focused her attention on her ailing tooth. After a while, she affirmed, *"I want my tooth to stop hurting me."* She continued to focus on the tooth, feeling the pain and going through it until she could see and feel the infected area clearly. She told us that she could feel distorted energy penetrating her tooth and knew it was the cause of her pain. She also told us that she was confident that she could remove the energy and make the pain go away. It was this confidence that compelled her to repeat the same affirmation over and over again like a mantra.

It didn't take long for sense of euphoria to engulf her and replace the pain and anxiety. To her child's mind, the process was so natural that she didn't tell anyone about what she'd done. Instead, once the pain was gone, she went outside to play.

The next morning, she decided to tell her father. But instead of being pleased, he told her that the healing wasn't real and that he would take her to the dentist the next day.

At the dentist's office, she was told that the healing was a coincidence, and not a result of anything a little girl had done.

Years passed, but the memory of what happened never faded. When she came to us, we quickly recognized that she had the uncanny ability to focus her mind and to muster large amounts of prana for healing. We encouraged her to begin healing once again and helped her create her own healing space, so that she could collect healing energy and focus it without blockages or distorted energy getting in the way.

## What is a Woman's Healing Space?

A woman's healing space is something she creates within her energy field. It's a place where a woman can use her healing skills to heal her body, soul, and spirit and to do the same for the people she loves.

To create your healing space, you will combine the energy and consciousness of two resource fields, the field of prakriti and the field of empathy. You already know that the field of prakriti is the primordial field of feminine energy. What you might not know is that the field of prakriti plays an important role in healing, because it's not readily subject to the distorted interactions that pollute other resource fields. This means that the prana emerging from the field of prakriti has fewer impurities. With fewer impurities, the energy will radiate more freely and it will have more power. So it will enhance a woman's ability to perform healing on both the physical level and on the subtle levels of energy and consciousness.

The field of empathy is another resource field that will enhance a woman's ability to heal. It has a powerful effect on a woman's relationship to herself and to other people. And it provides a medium through which energy can be exchanged selflessly without the "I" or the ego getting in the way.

By centering yourself in the field of empathy, you will create a compassionate healing space where you and your patients can meet energetically.

The field of empathy has three parts. The three parts are the public field of empathy, the personal field of empathy, and the transcendent field of empathy.

To create your healing space in order to heal yourself, heal other people, or heal your relationship to the source of healing, you must center yourself in the field of prakriti and the appropriate field of empathy. To use your healing space to heal yourself, you will center yourself in the personal field of empathy. To use your healing space to heal other people, you will center yourself in the public field of empathy. And to use your healing space to heal your relationship to the source of healing, you will center yourself in the transcendent field of empathy.

In the exercise that follows, you will create your healing space by centering yourself in your field of prakriti and your three fields of empathy.

---

## Exercise: Creating Your Healing Space

To create your healing space, find a comfortable position with your back straight. Close your eyes and breathe deeply through your nose for two to three minutes. Then count backward from five to one and from ten to one. Use the Standard Method to relax your muscles and to center yourself in your authentic mind. Then assert, *"It's my intent to center myself in my prakriti field."* Continue by asserting, *"It's my intent to turn my organs of perception inward on the level of my prakriti field."* Take a moment to enjoy the shift. Then assert, *"It's my intent to center myself in my three fields of empathy."* Continue by asserting, *"It's my intent to turn my organs of perception inward on the level of my three fields of empathy."* Take about fifteen minutes to enjoy your healing space. Then bring yourself out of the meditation by counting from one to five. Repeat as needed.

By centering yourself in the prakriti field and your three fields of empathy you will create a healing space. By returning to it regularly and by strengthening it through "resonating," your healing space will become a safe haven where you can access the energy you need to heal yourself, other people, and your relationship to the source of healing.

## Exercise: Resonating to Enhance Your Healing Space

To maintain your healing space, you must keep it strong and free from distorted energy. To do that, we've included an exercise called resonating. When used regularly, resonating will strengthen your healing space so that you can muster more prana for healing.

Resonating can be practiced almost anywhere you can make audible sounds without being disturbed. To perform resonating, sit in a comfortable position with your back straight. Close your eyes and breathe deeply through your nose for two to three minutes. Then count backward from five to one and from ten to one. Use the Standard Method to relax your muscles and to center yourself in your authentic mind. Then assert, *"It's my intent to center myself in my prakriti field."* Take a few moments to enjoy the shift. Then assert, *"It's my intent to center myself in my field of empathy."* Continue by asserting, *"It's my intent to fill my prakriti field with prana."* Then assert, *"It's my intent to fill my field of empathy with prana."* When you're ready to resonate, inhale into your healing space, and when you exhale, chant ohm.

Ohm, in Sanskrit, is the sound of the universal vibration. This is the sound uttered by the universe at the moment of creation. It's also the sound of the life force that continues to animate all living beings.

As you chant ohm, feel the energy in your healing space grow stronger. After a short time, you will feel that you're sinking deeper into your healing space. Surrender to the feeling and allow the prana from your healing space to radiate through your physical body and energy field. In a short time you will feel that the ohm you're chanting has become the singular expression of what you're experiencing and feeling. It's not necessary to chant too loudly, but it is best when you chant audibly. Continue chanting for about ten minutes. After ten minutes, bring yourself out of the exercise by counting from one to five.

The effects of resonating, especially after you've been doing it for a few days or weeks, will be profound. Resonating will enhance the size of your healing space. And by radiating prana from the fields of empathy you will be able to perform healing safely and with growing confidence.

Once you've created your healing space and you've begun to strengthen it through resonating, you're ready to learn a simple technique that you can reliably use for healing

## Exercise: Healing Yourself

In the exercise that follows, you will use your healing space to heal yourself. You can heal a physical condition or a pattern you wish to overcome. Once you've made your choice, sit in a comfortable position with your back straight. Then close your eyes and breathe deeply through your nose for two to three minutes. Count backward from five to one and from ten to one. Then use the Standard Method to relax your muscles and to center yourself in your authentic mind. When you're ready to continue, assert, *"It's my intent to center myself in my prakriti field."* Then assert, *"It's my intent to turn my organs of perception inward on the level of my prakriti field."* Continue by asserting, *"It's my intent to fill my prakriti field with prana."* Take a few moments to enjoy the shift. Then assert, *"It's my intent to center myself in my personal field of empathy."* Continue by asserting, *"It's my intent to turn my organs of perception inward on the level of my personal field of empathy."* Next assert, *"It's my intent to fill my personal field of empathy with prana."* Take a few moments to enjoy the shift. Then assert, *"It's my intent that healing energy flows through my healing space into the area of my body I've chosen to heal."* Don't do anything after that. Just enjoy the process. Take fifteen minutes to perform the healing. After fifteen minutes visualize that the body part you chose to heal is glowing with radiant good health. Then count from one to five. When you reach the number five, open your eyes and bring yourself out of the exercise. Repeat as needed.

In the next exercise you will use your healing space to heal another person. It's important to note that when you perform healing on another person, it's essential to get their permission first and that you explain what you will be doing physically and energetically.

## Exercise: Healing Another Person

To heal another person, sit in a comfortable position with your back straight. Choose the condition you want to heal and keep it in mind.

Then close your eyes and breathe deeply through your nose for two to three minutes. Count backward from five to one and from ten to one. Then use the Standard Method to relax your muscles and to center yourself in your authentic mind. When you're ready to continue, assert, *"It's my intent to center myself in my prakriti field."* Then assert, *"It's my intent to turn my organs of perception inward on the level of my prakriti field."* Continue by asserting, *"It's my intent to fill my prakriti field with prana."* Take a few moments to enjoy the shift. Then assert, *"It's my intent to center myself in my public field of empathy."* Continue by asserting, *"It's my intent to turn my organs of perception inward on the level of my public field of empathy."* Next assert, *"It's my intent to fill my public field of empathy with prana."* Take a few moments to enjoy the shift. Then assert, *"It's my intent to create a visual screen eight feet (two-and-a-half meters) in front of me."* Continue by asserting, *"It's my intent to visualize the person I want to heal on the screen in front of me."* As soon as the person appears on the screen assert, *"It's my intent that healing energy flows from my healing space into the area of my client's body I've chosen to heal."* Don't do anything after that. The prana emerging from your healing space will flow into the body parts that need it most. Continue the process for fifteen minutes. After fifteen minutes, visualize that the body part you chose to heal is glowing with radiant good health. Then release your client and the visual screen. Count from one to five next. When you reach the number five, open your eyes and bring yourself out of the exercise. Repeat as needed.

## Exercise: Healing Your Relationship to the Source of Healing

The source of healing goes by many names. But what you call it doesn't affect your relationship to it. In this exercise you will use your healing space to enhance your relationship to the source of healing. This will make you a more effective healer and will enhance your experience of transcendence. To begin the process, sit in a comfortable position with your back straight. Then close your eyes and breathe deeply through your nose for two to three minutes. Count backward from five to one and from ten to one. Then use the Standard Method to relax your muscles and to center yourself in your authentic mind. When you're ready to continue, assert, *"It's my intent to center myself in my prakriti field."* Then assert, *"It's my intent to turn my organs of perception inward on the level of my prakriti field."* Continue by asserting, *"It's my intent to fill my prakriti field with prana."* Take a few moments to enjoy the shift. Then assert, *"It's my intent to center myself in my transcendent field of empathy."* Continue by asserting, *"It's my intent to turn my organs of perception inward on the level of my transcendent field of empathy."* Continue by asserting, *"It's my intent that the source of healing radiates its healing energy and consciousness through my body, soul, and spirit."* Don't do anything after that. Just enjoy the process. After fifteen minutes, count from one to five. When you reach the number five, open your eyes and bring yourself out of the exercise. Repeat as needed.

## Menstruation and the Power of the Blood

In many parts of the world, it's believed that the source of a woman's healing power is in her menstrual blood. As long as a woman bled, this power could be used to create children. And it could be used to heal the sick, and to heal relationships that had been poisoned by projections of distorted energy and karmic baggage.

In the Bon tradition, the indigenous culture of Tibet that preceded the introduction of Buddhism, it was believed that the Earth Goddess gave menstrual blood to women to use in healing. That energy could then be used as a form of medication to heal, and to fertilize plants (Pröll 2004).

In Mesopotamia, it was believed that the great Goddess Ninhursag created men from clay and gave them her "blood of life."

The Gnostics adopted some of these ideas and used menstrual blood in their rituals until the seventh century when all rituals involving the menstrual blood were forbidden by the Church.

Science has validated the healing properties of menstrual blood. Researchers recently found that menstrual blood is highly oxygenated and that cells taken from menstrual blood can be cultivated and used like stem cells to repair damaged heart tissue.

In a recent Japanese experiment, Dr. Shunichiro Miyoshi, a cardiologist at Keio University School of Medicine in Tokyo, and colleagues, had nine volunteers donate menstrual blood. From this blood, scientists harvested the precursor cells called mesenchymal cells (MMCs).

After being put together in a culture with cells from the hearts of rats, about 20 per cent of MMCs began beating spontaneously and eventually formed sheets of heart muscle tissue.

According to a report by AFP news agency, this success rate is about a hundred times higher than the 0.2 to 0.3 percent success of stem cells derived from human bone marrow (Miyoshi).

Even though it's clear, at least to medical researchers, that a woman's menstrual blood has healing properties, in many societies people continue to fear its power. This irrational fear is nothing new.

Saint Hieronymus, a Christian cleric who lived in the seventh century, wrote: "Nothing is as impure as a woman during her period; whatever she touches becomes impure." These views were so widely accepted by the church that, in the seventh century, women were not allowed to enter a church if they were menstruating (St. Heironymus).

## The Power of the Blood

Things are different now. Medical research has validated the fact that a woman who menstruates regularly is healthy and that her body goes through a process of detoxification and cell regeneration. From an energetic perspective, menstruation is a reflection of the cycle of creation and regeneration. The uterus's ability to keep and to give reflects the special relationship women have to both the universal feminine and to the earth that nourishes their body, soul, and spirit.

This means that it's time to recognize that a woman is more than an individual; she is a vortex through which the life force is channeled into the world, and through which the world is nourished and healed. This is a role every woman should cherish.

Unfortunately, despite all the positive aspects of menstruation, many women still see this time as a burden and an impediment to modern life, sometimes painful and often accompanied with uncomfortable symptoms.

We believe that a radiant woman should detach herself from this outmoded view of menstruation and liberate the power of the menstrual blood. To facilitate that process, we've developed an exercise called the Cycle of Life Meditation. The Cycle of Life Meditation is designed to help women overcome the negative feelings and thoughts associated with menstruation and to recognize that the menstrual cycle is a manifestation of a woman's power, creativity, and radiance.

## Exercise: The Cycle of Life Meditation

To begin the Cycle of Life Meditation, lie down on your back with your eyes closed. Breathe deeply through your nose for two to three minutes. Then count backward from five to one and from ten to one. Use the Standard Method to relax your muscles and to center yourself in your authentic mind. Then bring your mental attention to your uterus. Become aware of the rhythm of keeping and rejecting within the mucosa of the uterus.

Once you can feel the rhythm, synchronize your breathing with it. Inhale while you keep and exhale while you reject. Then assert, *"It's my intent to activate my lower physical material chakra."* As soon as the chakra has become activate, you will become aware that you have the power to accept life-affirming energy through the chakra and the power to reject distorted energy that blocks it.

After you've recognized that you have the power to accept and reject, assert, *"It's my intent to accept the life-affirming power in my menstrual blood and release the distorted energy from my uterus and vagina that blocks it."*

Almost immediately you will sense that your femininity has taken on a new dimension with more nuances and complexity. Enjoy the process for ten minutes. Then count from one to five and bring yourself out of the meditation. Repeat as needed.

## Summary

In this chapter you learned to enhance your healing power by creating your own healing space. Then you learned to use your healing space to heal yourself, other people, and your relationship to the source of healing. After that you learned to liberate the power of your menstrual blood by performing the Cycle of Life Meditation.

In the following chapter you will learn how to make the transition from a traditional relationship to a transcendent relationship. To make that transition you will learn to center yourself in your third heart field. Then you will learn exercises that will enable you to develop a transcendent relationship with your self, with your partner, and with your children.

# FOURTEEN

## *Transcendent Relationship*

A woman's power, creativity, and radiance are meant to be shared with the people she loves. In this chapter we will show you how you can share them all through transcendent relationship, first with yourself, then with your partner and children.

From the study of tantra, we learn that the divine couple Shakti-Shiva serves as the archetype for transcendent relationship. They're able to participate in transcendent relationship because they share energy and consciousness with one another freely.

It's Shakti's energy in the form of prana that breaks down the barriers that make people feel separate. And it's prana in combination with consciousness that transports people into transcendent relationship with one another.

Like an ancient tantric adept, you can use the prana and consciousness radiating through your energy field to transform your relationships. To do that, you must do two things. First you must stop indulging in destructive patterns that block your experience of transcendence. Second, you must learn to center yourself in your third heart field, because it's through the third heart field that you will experience transcendent relationship with yourself and with the people you love. Before you begin, however, it will be useful to look into what differentiates a transcendent relationship from a traditional relationship.

## From Traditional to Transcendent

When viewed from the outside, a traditional relationship and a transcendent relationship look virtually the same. Partners can live together, have children, and participate in the social and economic life of the community.

However, in traditional relationships women are expected to support their husbands, sacrifice their own needs for the sake of their loved ones, and transmit the core values of their society to their children. Unfortunately, even in the twenty-first century, restrictive beliefs and self-limiting archetypes are still being transmitted to children through the acculturation process.

That's not to say that a traditional relationship can't satisfy people. In some cases, it can because family members can still share pleasure, love, and intermittent intimacy with one another. However, the final goal of permanent intimacy and joy, which family members share in a transcendent relationship, will remain a distant dream.

That's why it's important to recognize that a traditional relationship is about living within limitations. In contrast, a transcendent relationship is about transcending limitations, which is why in a transcendent relationship a radiant woman will experience a satisfaction unavailable to women in traditional relationships.

## Seven Things You Must Stop Doing

To achieve a transcendent relationship, you must stop indulging in seven destructive patterns. All seven have one important feature in common. They will prevent you from enjoying a transcendent relationship with yourself, your partner, and your children.

The seven patterns are listed below. Under each pattern, you will find a simple exercise that you can use to overcome it. If you're stuck in any one of the patterns listed below, practice the exercise we've provided until the pattern no longer disturbs you.

### Pattern 1—Putting Yourself Down

In order to overcome the impulse to put yourself down, find a comfortable position with your back straight. Breathe deeply through your nose for two to three minutes. Then count backward from five to one and from ten to one. Use the Standard Method to relax your muscles and to center yourself in your authentic mind. Then assert, *"It's my intent to activate my first chakra."* Continue by asserting, *"It's my intent to center myself in my first chakra field."* Take a moment to enjoy the shift. Then use the thumb of your positive hand, right hand if you're right-handed and left hand if you're left-handed, to activate the acupuncture point in the back of your head. The acupuncture point is located in the back of your skull at the point where a bulge connects your head to the back of your neck.

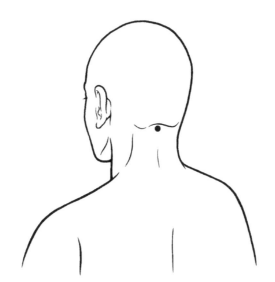

*Figure 19: The Acupuncture Point on the Back of the Neck*

By activating this acupuncture point, you will draw prana up from the governor meridian. The enhanced flow of prana will stimulate the seven traditional chakras mmbedded in the governor meridian. That will enhance your insight and intuition and make you feel more confident. It will also enhance the production of endorphins, which are associated with feelings of euphoria.

Stay centered in your first chakra field and maintain pressure on the acupuncture point for ten minutes. By activating the appropriate energy centers (acupuncture point and chakras), you will liberate the energy in your energy field that enhances self-worth and self-esteem. Practice the exercise regularly, and in a short time, you will stop putting yourself down.

### Pattern 2—Sacrificing Your Surface Boundaries

Your surface boundaries are the surfaces of your energy fields. They surround all of your energy fields (auras and resource fields) and your energetic vehicles (see figure 7). A woman with weak boundaries will feel insecure and won't be able to fully manifest the universal qualities of the feminine.

To strengthen your surface boundaries find a comfortable position with your back straight. Then breathe deeply through your nose for two to three minutes. Count backward from five to one and from ten to one. Use the Standard Method to relax your muscles and to center yourself in your authentic mind. Then assert, *"It's my intent to create a visual screen eight feet (two-and-a-half meters) in front of me."* Continue visualizing someone on the screen who doesn't respect your boundaries. It could be a demanding boss or a controlling family member. As soon as the person appears perform the No Mudra.

The No Mudra is designed to strengthen your resolve so that you can maintain strong boundaries. To perform the No Mudra use your thumbs and index fingers of both hands to form two loops that are connected to one another—like two links of a chain. Next, bring the tips of your middle fingers, ring fingers, and pinkies together so that they resemble the sides of a triangle.

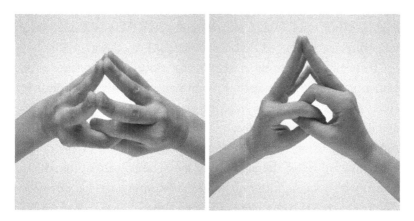

*Figure 20: The No Mudra*

Continue to hold the mudra while in a clear voice you assert, *"No"* to the person on the screen for five minutes, or until they no longer intrude into your personal space. Then release the mudra, the person on the screen and the visual screen. Bring yourself out of the exercise by counting from one to five. Repeat as needed.

## Pattern 3—Comparing Yourself to Others

You're a radiant woman, with access to all the prana and consciousness you need to succeed in your work and relationships.

Therefore it makes no sense to compare yourself to others. None-theless, if you continuously compare yourself to others and fall short or feel that you have to be perfect in order to feel good about yourself, then find a comfortable position with your back straight and close your eyes. Breathe deeply through your nose for two to three minutes. Then use the Standard Method to relax your muscles and to center yourself in your authentic mind. To continue, assert, *"It's my intent to activate my third chakra."* Then assert, *"It's my intent to center myself in my third chakra field."* Once you're centered in your third chakra field, perform alternate nostril breathing for ten minutes.

Alternate nostril breathing is an ancient yogic technique that will enhance your stability and self-awareness. It's these two qualities that will overcome your need to compare yourself to others.

To begin alternate nostril breathing, close your right nostril with your right thumb and inhale through your left nostril. Continue for a count of five. Then close your left nostril with your right ring finger and little finger, and at the same time, remove your thumb from the right nostril. Exhale through your right nostril for a count of eight. Next, inhale through the right nostril for a count of five. Close the right nostril with your right thumb and exhale through the left nostril for a count of eight. This completes one full round.

For the first two weeks, perform three rounds. After two weeks add one round per week until you're performing a maximum of seven rounds.

Alternate nostril breathing shouldn't be practiced if your nasal passages are blocked. And, under no circumstances should anything be forced. Repeat the exercise until the pattern no longer disturbs you.

### Pattern 4—Giving Away Personal Responsibility

If you've given away personal responsibility to someone else or to an outside institution, it's time to take it back. To do that, stand in front of a mirror and assert ten times, *"I'm in control of my energy field and I take personal responsibility for what I do."* After the tenth repetition, rub your hands together to polarize them. Then place your feminine hand, right hand if you're right-handed, left hand if you're left-handed, three inches (ten centimeters) above your heart chakra. Then place your masculine hand three inches (about seven-and-a-half centimeters) above your sixth chakra. Hold them there until you feel that the energy from both chakras has created a large field of prana that interpenetrates your energy field. As soon as the field emerges into your awareness, assert, *"It's my intent to center myself in the field of prana I've just created."* Then assert, *"It's my intent to turn my organs of perception inward on the field of prana I've just created."* Take ten minutes to enjoy the changes you feel physically and energetically. Then count from one to five and bring yourself out of the exercise. Repeat until the pattern no longer disturbs you.

*Pattern 5—Taking Everything Personally*

Women who take everything personally have problems with their personal rights. Your personal rights are regulated by your heart chakra. In many societies it's quite common for a woman to have her personal rights disrupted in childhood when a family member, or person in authority, violates her energetically.

In the exercise that follows, you will take back your personal rights. To do that, you will cut two pieces of paper into disks a foot and a half (half meter) in diameter. Color one side of each disk bright emerald green. It's important to color the circles yourself and fill both circles with pigment.

Once you've completed the first task, place one disk on the floor, with the color facing upward. Then lie down on it so that the center of the disk is centered on the back of your heart chakra. Place the other disk with the color facing your chest on the front of your heart chakra.

The disk below you will enhance the flow of prana up your back. The disk on the front will enhance the flow of prana down your front.

After you've placed the disks in the appropriate positions, close your eyes and breathe deeply through your nose for two to three minutes. Then count backward from five to one and from ten to one. Use the Standard Method to relax your muscles and to center yourself in your authentic mind. Then assert, *"It's my intent to activate my fourth chakra."* Continue by asserting, *"It's my intent to center myself in my fourth chakra field."* Stay centered in your fourth chakra field while you repeat this mantra to yourself in words, not thoughts, for five minutes: *"I will no longer take everything personally."* After repeating the mantra for five minutes, enjoy the changes you feel for another ten minutes. Then count from one to five and bring yourself out of the meditation. Repeat until the pattern no longer disturbs you.

*Pattern 6—Minimizing Your Strengths*

Most men have difficulty accepting their weaknesses. Most women have difficulty accepting their strengths. In order to accept yourself as the powerful, competent woman you are you will enhance the pressure in your energy system by activating your first and seventh chakras. Then you will perform the Self-Acceptance Mudra.

To begin, find a comfortable position with your back straight. Close your eyes and breathe through your nose for two to three minutes. Then count backward from five to one and from ten to one. Use the Standard Method to relax your muscles and to center yourself in your authentic mind. Then assert, *"It's my intent to activate my first chakra."* Continue by asserting, *"It's my intent to center myself in my first chakra field."* Take a few moments to enjoy the shift. Then assert, *"It's my intent to activate my seventh chakra."* Continue by asserting, *"It's my intent to center myself in my seventh chakra field."* Take a few moments to enjoy the shift. Then open your eyes and perform the Self-Acceptance Mudra.

To perform the mudra, bring your tongue to your top palate and slide it back until the hard palate curls upward and softens. Keep the tip of your tongue in contact with your upper palate while you place the soles of your feet together. Next, bring the mounts of Venus and the edges of your thumbs together. Then slide your right index finger over your left index finger so that the tip of the right finger rests atop the second joint of your left finger. The middle fingers are placed together so that the tips are touching. Once they're touching, place the outsides of the ring fingers together from the first to the second joint. Then bring the inside of the pinkies together from the tips to the first joints. After ten minutes, release the mudra. Then count from one to five and bring yourself out of the exercise. Repeat until the pattern no longer disturbs you.

### Pattern 7—Self-Sabotage

A woman can sabotage herself in her family life, work, and relationships, even her relationship to herself, when she has a third chakra blockage. A third chakra blockage will make a woman feel insecure in all her interactions. It will disrupt self-trust, satisfaction, and the sense of belonging. Unfortunately, third chakra blockages are quite common for women living in modern society.

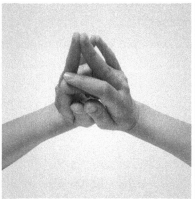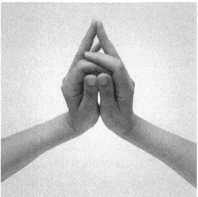

*Figure 3 (repeated): The Self-Acceptance Mudra*

In order to overcome the pattern of self-sabotage and the third chakra blockage that supports it, cut a piece of paper into a circle a foot and a half in diameter (half meter). Then color or paint one side yellow. The yellow should be bright and clear. It's important to color the circle yourself and fill the whole circle with pigment.

Once you've completed the first task, sit down on a straight-backed chair, in a quiet place where you won't be disturbed. Then place the circle under your bare feet, with the colored side facing upward. Close your eyes and breathe deeply through the nose for two to three minutes. Then count backward from five to one and from ten to one next. Use the Standard Method to relax your muscles and to center yourself in your authentic mind. Then assert, *"It's my intent to activate my third chakra."* Continue by asserting, *"It's my intent to center myself in my third chakra field."* Finally assert, *"It's my intent that the energy radiating from the yellow disk fills my third chakra field with satisfaction, security, and the feeling that I belong."*

Take fifteen minutes to enjoy the meditation. Then count from one to five. When you reach the number five, open your eyes and bring yourself out of the exercise. Repeat the exercise until the pattern no longer disturbs you.

## Exercise: Transcendent Relationship with Yourself

Now that you've learned to overcome the seven patterns that interfere with transcendent relationship, you're ready to experience transcendent relationship with yourself. To do that, you will perform the Third Heart Field Meditation. In the Third Heart Field meditation you will center yourself in your third heart field while you will perform the Orgasmic Bliss Mudra.

Your third heart field is a resource field that radiates bliss through your energy field and physical body. It's called the third heart field because of its connection to your first heart (human heart) and your second heart (heart chakra). The Orgasmic Bliss Mudra is designed to bring bliss emerging from Atman into your consciousness awareness. Atman is the thumb-sized point at the right side of your heart where bliss emerges into your conscious awareness.

By centering yourself in your third heart field and performing the Orgasmic Bliss Mudra, you will become the observer of the movie of your mind. Restrictive beliefs and taboos that once limited your freedom will melt away, and intimacy and joy will become permanent aspects of your life and relationships.

To perform the Third Heart Field Meditation, find a comfortable position with your back straight. Close your eyes and breathe deeply through your nose for two to three minutes. Then count backward from five to one and from ten to one. Use the Standard Method to relax your muscles and to center yourself in your authentic mind. Then assert, *"It's my intent to center myself in my third heart field."* Continue by asserting, *"It's my intent to turn my organs of perception inward on the level of my third heart field."* Take two to three minutes to enjoy the shift.

Then open your eyes and keep them slightly unfocused. While you remain centered in your third heart field, perform the Orgasmic Bliss Mudra.

To perform the mudra, place the tip of your tongue on your upper palate. Then bring it straight back until it comes to rest at the point where the hard palate rolls up and becomes soft. Once the tip of your tongue is in that position, put the bottom of your feet together so that the soles are touching. Then bring your hands in front of your solar plexus, with the inside tips of your thumbs together.

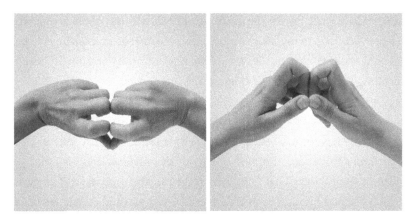

*Figure 9 (repeated): The Orgasmic Bliss Mudra*

Continue by bringing the outside of your index fingers together, from the tips to the first joint. Next, bring the outside of your middle fingers together, from the first to the second joint. The fourth and fifth fingers should be curled into your palm.

After your tongue, fingers, and feet are in position, close your eyes and enjoy the exercise for ten more minutes. Then release the mudra and bring yourself out of the meditation by counting from one to five.

You may experience lightness or the sensation that you're floating inside your energy field during or after the exercise. Don't be alarmed by either sensation. There is nothing wrong. Both the lightness and the floating sensation indicate that the life force is penetrating more deeply into your energy field and that you're transforming your relationship to your self.

If you practice the exercise daily for as little as a week, you will experience the benefits that come from having a transcendent relationship with yourself.

## Transcendent Relationship with Your Partner

Once you've experienced transcendent relationship with yourself, the next step is to experience transcendent relationship with your partner. However, before you can experience transcendent relationship with your male partner, you must be able to overcome one last hurdle. You must be able to love male power. That can be difficult because, even in the twenty-first century, many woman love men but resent or even reject male power. Fortunately, you can overcome any animosity you might have by creating the mutual field of prana with your partner.

## Creating the Mutual Field of Prana

It's not widely known, even among people seeking transcendence, that partners can create a field of energy with universal qualities that surrounds them both. That field, which we call the mutual field of prana, will be strong enough to prevent karmic baggage and restrictive beliefs from interfering with their experience of intimacy.

Now here's the best part: the mutual field of prana will continue to connect partners together, so that they can share pleasure, love, intimacy, and joy even when they're separated from one another by great distances or for long periods of time.

To create the mutual field of prana, you and your partner will sit, facing each other, eight feet (two and a half meters) apart. Once you're in position close your eyes and breathe deeply through the nose for two to three minutes. When you're ready to continue, count backward from five to one and from ten to one. Then use the Standard Method to relax your muscles and to center yourselves in your authentic mind. When you're ready to continue, assert, *"It's my intent to activate my thirteen chakras in body space."* Once your chakras are active, assert, *"It's my intent to center myself in the chakra fields of my thirteen chakras in body space."* Continue by asserting, *"It's my intent to fill my thirteen chakra fields in body space with prana."* Take a few moments to enjoy the shift. Then assert, *"It's my intent to create a mutual field of prana by radiating prana to my partner from my thirteen chakras in body space."* Don't do anything after that. Just let the energy radiate freely for ten minutes. After ten minutes, bring yourselves out of the exercise by counting from one to five. Repeat the exercise until you can share prana without anger or resentment getting in the way.

## Exercise: Transcendent Relationship with Your Partner

Once you've learned to create the mutual field of prana with your partner, you're ready to make the transition to a transcendent relationship. To do that, you and your partner will center yourselves in your third heart field and perform the Orgasmic Bliss Mudra. Then you will let the bliss emerging through your third heart transform your relationship to each other.

To begin the exercise, sit facing each other with your backs straight, eight feet (two-and-a-half meters) apart. Then close your eyes and breathe deeply through your nose for two to three minutes. Count backward from five to one and from ten to one. Then use the Standard Method to relax your muscles and to center yourselves in your authentic mind. Continue by asserting, *"It's my intent to center myself in my third heart field."* To enhance the effect, assert, *"It's my intent to turn my organs of perception inward on the level of my third heart field."* Take two to three minutes to enjoy the shift. Then perform the Orgasmic Bliss Mudra (see the exercise above). Hold the mudra for five minutes. Then assert, *"It's my intent that bliss transforms my relationship to my partner."* Don't do anything after that. Just enjoy the process for another ten minutes while you continue to hold the mudra. After ten minutes, release the mudra and bring yourselves out of the meditation by counting from one to five.

If you and your partner practice this exercise together daily for at least a week, you will begin to experience the benefits that come from a transcendent relationship.

## Transcendent Relationship with Your Children

A transcendent relationship with your child can begin in the womb. That's because even a preborn child has a fully developed consciousness, which means it reacts to its physical and energetic environment.

New clinical research from Dr. Wendy Ann McCarthy indicates that

> We are conscious and aware, learning intensely and actively, com-
> municating and forming relationships from the beginning of life.
> Our earliest experiences in the womb, during birth and as young
> babies profoundly shape and set in motion physical, mental, emo-
> tional and relationship life patterns that can be life enhancing or
> diminishing. (McCarthy 2013, 21–22)

A pregnant woman can enhance her relationship to her preborn child
by creating a healthy energetic bond with it while it's growing in her
womb. This not only benefits the child; it benefits the mother. By enhancing energetic interactions with her preborn child, a mother is less
likely to experience postpartum depression or have karmic blockages
interfere with the free flow of prana between her energy field and the
energy field of her developing child.

---

### Exercise: Bonding Exercise for the Preborn

With this in mind we've created the Preborn Bonding Meditation. A
woman can begin practicing this meditation at the beginning of the
second trimester.

To begin the meditation, find a comfortable place where you won't
be disturbed. Then lie down on your back and bring your attention to
the minor energy centers in your palms. Inhale into the energy centers
in your palms to activate them. On the exhalation, chant ohm from
your heart chakra. Your heart chakra resonates in C in the major musical scale. By chanting ohm from your heart chakra, you will create a
sympathetic vibration that activates the energy centers in your palms
even more.

After chanting for two to three minutes, place your palms on your
abdomen with your fingers facing each other. Continue chanting from
your heart chakra and let the vibration created by your chanting create
a healthy and enduring energetic connection to your preborn child.

Continue for ten more minutes. Then remove your hands and bring yourself out of the meditation by counting from one to five. Repeat once a day as long as you're pregnant.

## Baby Massage

Once you've given birth you can enrich your energetic bond with your newborn by giving it a baby massage. A baby massage provides your newborn with a sense of security and belonging. It also strengthens its immunological system. Babies who are touched and massaged regularly become more self-confident and sleep better. The child's motor skills improve, he or she develops a more expressive personality, and her or she can empathize more deeply with the feelings of others. A baby massage does all this by enhancing the flow of prana through the baby's energy field and between the baby and its mother.

Before you begin a baby massage, it's important to remember to warm the room and the oil you will be using for the massage. Avoid oil that is too thick or has a strong odor. And most important, always massage your baby with flat palms.

---

## Exercise: Baby Massage

When you're ready to begin, lay the baby on your lap on its front. Then rub your hands together to polarize them. Next, touch your baby's feet with your palms. Sense your baby's reaction. Does she or he enjoy what you're doing? Not all babies enjoy being massaged. By checking your baby's reaction you can determine if you have the baby's permission to proceed.

After rubbing your baby's feet, rub the back of the legs. Then place your hands opposite one another, in the middle of your baby's back, an inch or two (two-and-a-half or five centimeters) from her or his spine. Avoid touching or massaging the spine directly. Instead, make two big circles with the flat of your hands on the right side and the left side of your baby's spine. Next, rub their right and left shoulders and arms.

Continue for three or four minutes. Then turn your baby over and rub the front of your baby's legs in a circle with flat palms. Rub her or his belly gently with the palms, making circles with your hands. Continue by rubbing your baby's chest and shoulders. Then rub your baby's arms and hands.

The whole process should take no more than ten minutes. After the massage rest alongside your baby and let the baby respond to the massage in its own individual way.

We recommend that you perform a baby massage with your newborn twice a week, at the same time each day.

## Exercise: Preschool Chanting

Once she or he is able to talk, you can chant with your child from your seven traditional chakras. This will enhance your energetic bond and enable you to develop a transcendent relationship with your child. To perform preschool chanting, sit facing your child. Gaze at your child while you freely radiate your pleasure and enjoyment. Then bring your mental attention to your first chakra and chant *ohm* in the tone of G.

G will create a sympathetic vibration in your first chakra the same way a sympathetic vibration is created in a violin string when a tuning fork, with the same tone, is struck next to it.

Raise the *ohm* one note for each chakra. A for the second chakra, B for the third chakra, C for the fourth chakra, D for the fifth chakra, E for the sixth chakra, and F for the seventh chakra.

If you're not sure what tone to chant, begin the exercise by chanting the lowest tone you can vocalize and then shift the tone until you feel that a sympathetic resonance is emerging from the first chakra. The sympathetic resonance, which will emerge as a vibration or glowing sensation, will indicate that you are chanting the appropriate tone. You can use the same technique to make sure you are chanting the appropriate tone for all seven traditional chakras.

In preschool chanting, you will chant the tone from your first chakra by yourself first. After you've finished chanting invite your child to chant the same tone with you two more times. Then raise the tone one note and chant three times from your second chakra along with your child.

Continue in the same way, raising the tone one note and chanting three times from the third, fourth, fifth, sixth, and seventh chakras together with your child. After you and your child have chanted from the seven traditional chakras, continue chanting from your heart chakras for another five minutes. Perform this exercise for as long as your child continues to enjoy it.

## Summary

In this chapter you learned to make the transition from a traditional relationship to a transcendent relationship. To experience a transcendent relationship with yourself you learned to overcome destructive patterns that blocked your experience of transcendence. And you learned to center yourself in your third heart field. To experience a transcendent relationship with your partner you learned to create the mutual field of prana and to share bliss. To create a transcendent relationship with your children you learned to bond with your preborn, to perform a baby massage, and to perform preschool chanting.

We've devoted our final chapter to healing the female spirit. In order to heal the female spirit you will learn to use self-limiting patterns to discover your personal dharma. Then you will learn to perform exercises to enhance the two most important elements of your female spirit: strength and love. After that you will learn to celebrate the universal qualities of the feminine.

# FIFTEEN
# Healing the Female Spirit

A young woman who has healed her spirit will become a beacon of radiance to those around her. She will share the universal qualities of the feminine effortlessly with her friends and family and use her discernment to judge the value of worldly things. Because she has self-esteem and experiences her authentic identity, no one will be able to control her or manipulate her. Her decisions will enhance her relationship to herself and to other people. Loving her body will be natural for her because she knows that it's the outer manifestation of the universal feminine. She won't sacrifice her innocence or personal power for a man. And she will wait patiently as her dharma unfolds. Then she will embrace it enthusiastically.

When an adult woman has healed her spirit she will choose a partner who honors her femininity and who doesn't stand above or below her. She will share her power, creativity, and radiance freely and provide a healthy environment for her family. She will take special care to nourish her children, while at the same time she participates in the worldly activities that nourish her and support her spiritual growth.

When a mature woman has healed her spirit she will experience a rich inner life. Because of that she won't fear death. Although she is elderly she will continue to love her body and will treat it with tenderness and respect. She will share her wisdom freely and help the young grow up with strength and dignity. Because she has healed her spirit, she will regret nothing, even her youthful mistakes. She will be respected by her peers because she will continue to embrace the universal qualities of the feminine in her body, soul, and spirit. And, as an elder, she will maintain the continuity of her community.

## A Woman's Spiritual Foundation

A woman who has healed her spirit at any stage of life will feel the same transcendent love and joy for herself that she feels for other people. Such a woman will have strength, self-knowledge, and will be free from worldly attachments.

Human love alone cannot heal your spirit, although for short periods it can be intoxicating. To heal your spirit it's necessary to build a strong foundation on the spiritual level. To do that, a woman must do three things. She must gain self-knowledge by finding her personal dharma. She must enhance her self-love, if necessary, so that she is free from worldly attachments. And, she must be able to share the two most important elements of her spirit, strength, and transcendent love (bliss).

We will begin our journey of spiritual healing by learning how a woman can find her personal dharma. The word dharma comes from the Sanskrit root *dhri*, meaning to "uphold" or to "sustain." Both yoga and tantra teach that all human beings share a collective dharma, which is to achieve self-realization. Every human being also has a personal dharma, which is their unique path of healing and personal liberation.

## Finding Your Personal Dharma

To find your personal dharma you will use your innate strengths and talents, your dominant karmic patterns, and the yearning of your third heart. The yearning of the third heart is the yearning for bliss, and the freedom that comes from knowing and following your dharma.

To begin the process, make a list of your most important talents and strengths. Talents and strengths can include strong nerves, a powerful body, strength of character, passion, empathy for others, and the talents associated with sport, art, music, and academia. In our work, we've found that the talents and strengths that bear directly on personal dharma emerge in childhood. They have a sense of reality about them, and they motivate a person to manifest their will, desire, and creativity in the world.

Once you've made a list of your talents and strengths, the next step will be to list your dominant karmic patterns.

## Your Dominant Karmic Patterns

Your dominant karmic patterns are the most compelling patterns you brought with you into this life. Most people have one dominant karmic pattern. Some people have as many as two or three. By limiting your access to your innate power, creativity, and radiance, and by frustrating your best efforts to know yourself these patterns motivate you to move forward and to heal yourself spiritually.

After you've listed your dominant karmic patterns, you will spin them in a positive direction, so that they serve as a guide to finding your personal dharma. In that way your self-limiting patterns will become self-liberating patterns.

To help you in this process we've included four of the most common self-limiting patterns in the list below. You can use our list as a basis for your own list. When making your list, try to be as honest and thorough as possible.

## Self-Limiting Patterns

1. Judgmental and intolerant
2. Controlling and manipulative
3. Self-destructive
4. Emotionally withholding

Once you've completed your list, it's important to resist the impulse to connect the patterns with negative feelings and then dwell on your inability to overcome them. Instead, spin your negative pattern in a positive direction. We can use the first pattern on our list, judgmental and intolerant, to illustrate how you can do that.

If you've engaged in this pattern, it indicates that your personal rights were lost or taken from you in a past life. So, an aspect of your personal dharma includes restoring your personal rights in this life.

The example above illustrates how you can spin a negative pattern in a positive direction. By doing that with all the patterns on your list, you will change your list of self-limiting patterns into list of self-liberating patterns.

We've spun all the patterns on our list, and included exercises that you can use to overcome them. You can use our list as a guide to making your list and healing the patterns that appear on it.

## Self-Liberating Patterns

### 1. Judgmental and Intolerant

This pattern indicates that your personal rights were lost or taken from you in a past life and that you must restore your personal rights in this life. To overcome this pattern activate your heart chakra, center yourself in your heart chakra field, and fill your heart chakra field with prana (go to chapter 3).

### 2. Controlling and Manipulative

This pattern indicates that you lost control of your energy field and physical body in a past life and that you must restore your personal power and self-control in this life. To do that, perform the Orgasmic Bliss Mudra (go to chapter 4), and while you hold the mudra, activate your heart chakra, then center yourself in your heart chakra field and fill it with prana (go to chapter 3).

### 3. Self-Destructive

This pattern indicates that in a past life you had such a negative self-image that you saw no other alternative than to ruin every good thing that the universe gave you. To overcome this pattern you must restore your authentic identity and self-esteem. To do that, you must heal your aspects of mind and release foreign aspects of mind from your subtle energy field. Then you must perform the Self-Esteem Mudra (go to chapter 5).

### 4. Emotionally Withholding

This pattern indicates that you were deprived of the right to express your emotions and feelings in a past life and that your personal rights must be restored in this life. To do that, activate your heart chakra. Center yourself in your heart chakra field and fill it with prana. Then activate your second through fifth chakras, center yourself in the corresponding chakra fields, and fill them with prana (go to chapter 3).

Once you've made your list of strengths and talents, and spun your self-limiting patterns into self-liberating patterns, you can combine the lists in order to uncover the essential elements of your personal dharma. For example if you have physical strength and have a passion for sports and your self-liberating pattern is to regain your personal power and self-control, your personal dharma could include becoming a sports physician, a physical trainer, or even someone who leads expeditions. The last thing you must do to find your personal dharma is to enhance the yearning of your third heart.

By enhancing the yearning of your third heart, you will validate what you've already learned about your dharma, and you will gain additional insights into how you can manifest it in the world.

### Exercise: Enhancing the Yearning of Your Third Heart

To enhance the yearning of your third heart, you must strengthen your will, desire, and transcendent love (bliss) and then combine them. To do that, find a comfortable position with your back straight. Close your eyes and breathe deeply through your nose for two to three minutes. Then count backward from five to one and from ten to one. Use the Standard Method to relax your muscles and to center yourself in your authentic mind.

Once you're centered, you're ready to combine your authentic will, desire, and unconditional love. To do that, assert, *"It's my intent to turn my organs of perception inward on the level of my core field and experience my authentic will."* Take a few moments to experience your authentic will. Then assert, *"It's my intent to turn my organs of perception inward on the level of my core field and experience my authentic desire."* Take another few moments to experience your authentic desire. Continue by asserting, *"It's my intent to turn my organs of perception inward on the level of my core field and experience transcendent love."* Take another few moments to experience transcendent love. Then assert, *"It's my intent to combine my authentic will, desire, and transcendent love."* Take five minutes to experience the shift that takes place once you've combined all three.

You may experience lightness or the sensation that you're floating inside your energy field. Don't be disturbed by either sensation. There is nothing wrong. Feeling lighter indicates that you're centered in universal qualities. The sensation that you're floating indicates that your personal will and desire have temporarily been freed from the influence of karmic baggage and external projections. Take five minutes more to enjoy the effects. Then continue the exercise by performing the Mudra for Orgasmic Bliss.

To perform the mudra, place the tip of your tongue on your upper palate. Then bring it straight back until it comes to rest at the point where the hard palate rolls up and becomes soft. Once the tip of your tongue is in that position, put the bottom of your feet together so that the soles are touching. Then bring your hands in front of your solar plexus, with the inside tips of your thumbs together.

Continue by bringing the outside of your index fingers together, from the tips to the first joint. Next, bring the outside of your middle fingers together, from the first to the second joint. The fourth and fifth fingers should be curled into your palm. After your tongue, fingers, and feet are in position, close your eyes once again and continue the exercise for ten more minutes.

After ten minutes, release the mudra. Then count from one to five. When you reach the number five, open your eyes. You'll be wide-awake and perfectly relaxed.

Practice the meditation every night for two weeks. Then ask yourself this question: What is my personal dharma and how should I manifest it in the world? Be prepared to get the answers you seek through dreams, insights, pictures, and impressions that give you the "knowing" that you've found your personal dharma and know how to manifest it.

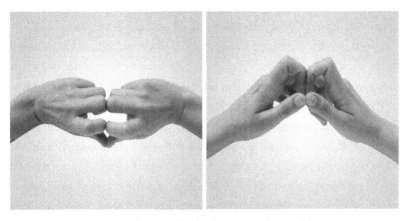

*Figure 9 (repeated): The Orgasmic Bliss Mudra*

Once you've discovered your personal dharma, you can use the knowledge and skill you gained from this book, along with your talents, strengths, and intuition to design a lifestyle and regimen of energy work that supports your dharma and is a celebration of the feminine spirit.

## Healing the Female Spirit

Now that you have the skills to find your personal dharma, the next step in healing your spirit will be to enhance its two most important elements, strength and love.

To do that, you will perform the Self-Love Meditation and the Light Body Field Meditation. In the Self-Love Meditation you will enhance your self-love by making the three forms of love—human love, spiritual love, and transcendent love—part of your life-affirming identity. In the Light Body Field Meditation you will center yourself in your light body field and add an additional step to the meditation you performed in chapter 12. After you've enhanced the essential qualities of the light body field, which are spiritual power and love, you will share them with the people you love.

---

### Exercise: Self-Love Meditation

Before you begin the Self-Love Meditation, it's important to recognize that self-love is more than feeling good about yourself. It's the recognition that you're a manifestation of the universal feminine, and that spiritual love is an essential part of your femininity and life-affirming identity.

To begin the Self-Love Meditation, find a comfortable position with your back straight. Close your eyes and breathe deeply through your nose for two to three minutes. Then count backward from five to one and from ten to one. Use the Standard Method to relax your muscles and to center yourself in your authentic mind. Then assert, *"It's my intent to visualize a screen eight feet (two-and-a-half meters) in front of me."* Continue by asserting, *"It's my intent to visualize myself on the screen with all of the universal qualities of the feminine radiating through me."* As soon as your image appears on the screen, assert, *"It's my intent to radiate human love to the image of myself on the screen from my human heart."* Continue by asserting, *"It's my intent to radiate unconditional love to the image of myself from my heart chakra."* Then assert, *"It's my intent to radiate transcendent love to the image of myself from Atman, my third heart."* Continue for five minutes. Then assert, *"It's my intent that the image of myself on the screen radiates love from her three hearts back to me."* Take ten minutes to experience the flow of love between you. Then release the image of yourself on the screen. Release the screen. Then bring yourself out of the meditation by counting from one to five. When you reach the number five, open your eyes. You'll feel wide-awake, perfectly relaxed, and better than you did before. Repeat as needed.

### Exercise: Light Body Field Meditation

To begin the Light Body Field Meditation, find a comfortable position with your back straight. Then close your eyes and breathe deeply through your nose for two to three minutes. Next, count backward from five to one and from ten to one. Use the Standard Method to relax your muscles and to center yourself in your authentic mind. Then assert, *"It's my intent to center myself in my light body field."* Continue by asserting, *"It's my intent to turn my organs of perception inward on the level of my light body field."* Take a few moments to enjoy the shift. Then assert, *"It's my intent to fill light body field with prana."* Enjoy the process for five minutes. Then assert, *"It's my intent to share the prana filling my light body field with the people I love."* Take fifteen minutes to experience the shift in your light body field as prana radiates through you. Then bring yourself out of the meditation by counting from one to five. When you reach the number five, open your eyes. You will feel wide-awake, perfectly relaxed, and better than you did before. Repeat as needed.

Now that you have the tools to heal your spirit and radiate it's strength and love freely, you're ready to celebrate the universal feminine. To do that, we've included three activities: the radiant woman's walk, the radiant woman's dance, and a woman's day of celebration. By performing these three activities, you will be able to celebrate the spirit of the universal feminine whenever you please.

## Exercise: The Radiant Woman's Walk

To perform the radiant woman's walk, find a pleasant location where you can walk without being disturbed. The woods or a secluded beach would be excellent choices. When you're ready, begin walking. As you walk, feel your feet making contact with the earth and the power of the universal feminine that emerges from it. If you stay focused, it won't be long before you feel a glowing sensation emerging from the minor energy centers in your feet.

As soon as you're aware of the glow, shift your attention to the minor energy centers in your hands. Continue to walk with your palms facing upward. Feel the minor energy centers in your hands make contact with the universal power of the feminine that interpenetrates the atmosphere. Once you feel a glowing sensation emerging from the minor energy centers in your hands, bring your attention to your heart chakra. Breathe into your heart chakra until it becomes active. Then assert, *"It's my intent to radiate prana from my heart chakra through my eyes, into the world around me."* Continue the radiant woman's walk for twenty minutes. In each step enjoy how the prana radiating through your eyes enriches your experience of the world.

## Exercise: The Radiant Woman's Dance

The radiant woman's dance can be performed with or without music. To begin, stand up straight with your shoulders back and head held high. Breathe deeply through your nose. As you breathe, feel that your breath and your emotions have become part of one radiant stream of energy. Continue breathing this way for five minutes. Then begin moving your right wrist. Move it in all directions, so that you feel that you're loosening the energetic knots that restrict its movement. Do the same with your left wrist. Then move your right elbow and your left elbow the same way. Next, move your shoulders and neck in all directions. Continue moving your right ankle, left ankle, right knee, left knee, right hip, left hip. Finally move your whole pelvis by moving your abdomen in all directions. After you've moved your pelvis in all directions and you feel the knots being released, begin to combine the movements you made with all your joints, so that you spontaneously perform the radiant woman's dance.

This is not a static dance, so move around, stop and start, change directions, and have fun. As your dance becomes more spontaneous more prana will pour through your energy field. This surge of prana will enable you to integrate your physical movements with your breath and emotions. Continue to dance for fifteen minutes.

During the radiant woman's dance, some women experience what can only be described as an energy orgasm. An energy orgasm, in contrast to a normal orgasm, emerges directly from your heart chakra. By synchronizing your physical movements with your feelings and breath, you will release vast amounts of prana. Prana vibrates and that vibration will penetrate your body to the deepest cellular level. From there it will expand and radiate through your whole body like an orgasm. If this surge of prana isn't blocked, it can bring you into a fuller recognition of the universal feminine and its ability to nourish you and heal you on the deepest levels of body, soul, and spirit.

## Exercise: Celebrating the Female Spirit

Another way to celebrate the universal qualities of the feminine is to experience a woman's day of celebration. A woman's day of celebration begins in the morning while you're still in bed. When you wake, remain in the region between sleep and wakefulness for as long as possible. In this state your brain wave frequency will be at the alpha-theta level. And you will experience your connection to the universal feminine before the problems of the world kick in to disturb you.

After you've experienced the alpha-theta level for a while get up and shower yourself. During your shower rinse your body with hot water. Pay special attention to any area that is tense. Then use the hot water to warm the area while you consciously breathe prana into it on each inhalation. Take your time. As soon as warmth has replaced tension rinse the area off with cold water. After you've completed your shower rub your body with a brush to improve your circulation.

Then dress in clothes that enhance your energy level. We suggest you dress in all natural fibers, and that the colors you choose make you feel good. Drink a cup of hot water next.

Then have a light breakfast with fresh foods that are full of prana. Fruit and whole grains would be a good choice. When you've finished breakfast, go for a walk in a natural environment.

Take frequent breaks to enjoy nature and to lean against the biggest trees you can find. Feel the prana emerging from each tree flowing through your body. If you're receptive, in a short time your organs of perception will become sharper and your experience of the natural environment will become more vivid.

You can increase your sensitivity to the natural environment and to the universal feminine by taking a swim in any natural body of water. Water is one of the five elements. And if you immerse yourself in a natural body of water, you will be able to feel prana invigorating your physical body and subtle energy field.

During your day of celebration, drink at least two-and-a-half quarts (three liters) of water. And after a healthy dinner of natural foods, watch the sun go down while you listen to your favorite classical music. Afterward take some time to review your day. Be aware of how negative feelings interfered with your ability to experience the universal qualities of the feminine in your body and in the world around you. Try to pinpoint where the negative feelings were located and which negative thoughts were attached to them. Then inhale into the body part where the negative feelings were located. Prana will enter the body part on each inhalation. When you exhale, let go of the negative feelings and thoughts and the tension in your body they created. Continue until all the tension in your body is released. Then relax and enjoy the rest of your day while you continue to celebrate the universal qualities of the feminine through your body, soul, and spirit.

By integrating the celebration of the female spirit into your life and relationships you will become an inspiration to both women and men. This is important because we believe it's time for every woman to take the next step in their personal journey, by creating a field of wellness and vitality that radiates through their auric fields and through the very cells of their body. In this way, they will become a vehicle of knowledge, femininity, and joy.

# Glossary

**Acupuncture point:** A subtle energy point located within a meridian.

**Ahamkara:** *Aspect of mind*; the decision maker; distills the information it receives from the other *aspects of mind* and uses it to create and/or support your perception of yourself and your relationships.

**Archetype bumping:** An exercise where you replace a self-limiting archetype you've integrated into your personality with a life-affirming archetype that enhances your power, creativity, and radiance.

**Aspects of mind:** Subtle energetic vehicles that serve as the foundation of your authentic identity. They are slightly larger than the physical body and come in four varieties—*manas, buddhi, chitta,* and *ahamkara*.

**Atman:** The third of the three hearts; a "thumb-sized" spot on the right side of your chest, where universal love in the form of bliss emerges into your conscious awareness. By following the Atman inward, you will become aware of your a priori union with Universal Consciousness.

**Attachments:** Energetic fields of distorted energy with individual qualities that can influence a woman's subtle energy field—and therefore her mind—in three ways: they can restrict a woman's access to prana, they can create restrictive patterns (personality issues) that are not an essential part of a woman's mind, and they can keep a woman attached to people and relationship issues that remain unresolved from childhood and/or past lives.

**Auric fields, auras:** Auric fields are large fields of prana that fill and surround your subtle energy field on each dimension. From the surface of your body on each dimension, your auric fields extend outward (in all directions) from about two inches (five centimeters) to more than twenty-six feet (six and a half meters). Structurally, each auric field is composed of an inner cavity and a thin surface boundary, which surrounds it and gives it its characteristic egg shape.

**Authentic desires:** Desires that come from your authentic mind. They help you stay centered in your subtle energy field and enhance the flow of prana through your subtle energy system.

**Authentic mind:** Composed of your energy field, your nervous system, and your organs of perception, which can be directed at both your external environment (the physical world) and your internal environment (the subtle worlds of energy and consciousness). It's your authentic vehicle of awareness and expression and your strong center in the subtle world of energy and consciousness.

**Bliss, orgasmic bliss:** The most powerful force in the universe. Every human being is in bliss—although most people are unaware of it. According to the tantrics, orgasmic bliss is an enduring condition, deep inside your energy field, created through the union of consciousness (Shiva) and energy (Shakti).

**Blockage:** Any field of energy with individual qualities which disrupts the flow of prana through the subtle energy field and which prevents a human being from remaining centered in their authentic mind.

**Boundaries:** Surfaces of the auras; composed of prana in the form of elastic fibers which criss-cross each other in every imaginable direction.

**Buddhi:** *Aspect of mind* that analyzes and compares an object, being and/or *energy field* that has been separated from its environment with what is already known. The *buddhi* allows you to put what it has studied into a specific context so that the *chitta* can confer a particular value on it.

**Chakra(s):** Sanskrit word which means "wheel." Chakras have two parts—the chakra field, which is an immense field of prana, and a gate that appears as brightly colored disk that spins rapidly at the end of what looks like a long axle or stalk. Chakras transmit and transmute *prana* into different frequencies for use by the *energetic vehicles* in your *energy field*; there are one hundred and forty six *chakras* within your *energy system*.

**Chakra healing:** A form of energetic healing in which prana emerging through the chakras is transferred to the area in the patient's body where it's needed most. By performing chakra healing, you can heal ailments in your body, mind and soul—as well as in your relationships, at their root, in your subtle energy field.

**Chao Yang:** The (two) Chao Yang meridians rise from a central point in the soles of the feet and pass through the outer sides of the ankles and legs where they connect with additional meridians at the base of the penis-vagina. Along with the two Chao Yin meridians they form minor energy centers in the feet.

**Chao Yin:** The two Chao Yin meridians rise from a central point in the soles of the feet and pass through the inside of the ankles and legs where they connect with additional meridians at the base of the penis-vagina. They are called negative leg channels because they are yin in relation to the Chao Yang meridians. Along with the two Chao Yang meridians they form minor energy centers in the feet.

**Character, good character:** Includes non-harming, discipline, courage, patience, perseverance, long suffering, and loyalty. These qualities can be enhanced in anybody who brings their subtle energy field into a state of radiant good health.

**Chitta:** *Aspect of mind*; confers a value on what has been isolated by *manas* and analyzed by *buddhi*.

**Cords:** Energetic projection of energy with individual qualities in the form of a long thin cord. It's a manifestation of dependency, need, and/or desire that can border on obsession. Cords manifest the perpetrator's desire or need to hold on to or have contact with his target.

**Dharma:** Comes from the Sanskrit root *dhri*, meaning to "uphold" or to "sustain." Both yoga and tantra teach that all human beings share a collective dharma which is to achieve self-realization. Every human being also has a personal dharma which is their unique path of healing and personal liberation. It's by following your dharma that you will learn who you are and what you are capable of achieving in this life.

**Dominant karmic patterns:** The most compelling patterns you brought with you into this life. Most people have one dominant karmic pattern. Some people have as many as two or three. By limiting your access to your innate power, creativity, and radiance—and by frustrating your best efforts to know yourself—these patterns motivate you to move forward and to heal yourself spiritually.

**Energetic blockage:** See blockage.

**Energetic projection:** Any projection of distorted energy with individual qualities. Projections can take the form of cords and can be accompanied by non-physical beings. When an energetic projection becomes trapped in a person's energy field it can cause self-limiting and anti-self patterns.

**Energetic vehicles:** There are two types of energetic vehicles in the human energy field—*energy bodies* and *sheaths*. Both are composed of *prana*; they serve as vehicles of awareness, cognition, assimilation, sensation, and expression—on each dimension of the physical and non-physical universe.

**Energy bodies:** Subtle bodies in the human energy field. They're composed entirely of energy with universal qualities. Functionally they allow you to be present in your energy field and experience the activities of the physical and non-physical universe via your awareness and your organs of perception.

**Energy system:** A system of subtle energetic organs composed of *chakras, meridians,* and *minor energy centers.* Your energy system supports your energy field. It can be thought of as a power plant and grid of sub-stations and power lines that transmute consciousness into *prana* and *prana* from one frequency into another.

**Energy with individual qualities:** Energy that evolves and involves through time-space. It can accumulate in your subtle energy field. Attachments to energy with individual qualities can disrupt the flow of prana through the subtle energy field and can prevent a person from being present.

**Energy with universal qualities:** Energy that never fundamentally changes. It goes by many names—shakti, prana, chi, etc. It's the energy that flows through your chakras and meridians. It emerges into a person's conscious awareness as pleasure, love, intimacy, and joy as well as truth, freedom, and bliss.

**Enlightenment:** A state of permanent bliss. In the state of enlightenment, the existential problem of existence disappears—and a person experiences a deep buzz of inner peace.

**Ever present now:** The eternal present; the space you inhabit when you are present in your authentic mind.

**External projections:** Energetic projections with individual qualities, which one person can project at another. Once you've become attached to an external projection, it will be integrated into your individual mind and ego and become part of the karmic baggage you carry in your energy field.

**Feminine energy:** After emerging from Universal Consciousness, creative feminine energy began to function as the driving force of evolution. It's feminine energy emerging from every corner of the universe and from every female of every species that provides the power to create and procreate. Feminine energy is universal and life-affirming. It motivates humans to unite and to experience intimacy with one another. And it enables them to experience a deeper liberation and joy.

**Field of empathy:** A resource field that will enhance a person's ability to heal. It provides a medium through which energy can be exchanged selflessly without the "I" or the ego getting in the way. The field of empathy has three parts—the public field of empathy, the personal field of empathy, and the transcendent field of empathy.

**Fragmentation:** Your energy field will become fragmented whenever an energetic vehicle has been ejected from it. The most common cause of fragmentation is the intrusion of distorted energy, with individual qualities, into your energy field.

**Functions of mind:** There are sixteen important functions of mind, in the core field, through which your power, creativity, and radiance emerge. They include intent, will, desire, resistance, surrender, acceptance, knowing, choice, commitment, rejection, faith, enjoyment, destruction, creativity, empathy, and love.

**Germ theory:** The brainchild of Louis Pasteur, who taught that it was the presence of microbes in the human body that caused disease. Once this new paradigm took root, the practice of medicine became more mechanical—and more divorced from a woman's healing space.

**Good character:** Includes non-harming, patience, perseverance, discipline, long suffering, and courage. Energy with universal qualities is both the foundation and product of good character. This means that people who have self-discipline and patience as well as courage—and who persevere in what they do—radiate prana freely and glow with inner beauty.

**Governor meridian:** The governor meridian is the most important masculine meridian in the human energy system. It originates at the perineum, at the base of the spine, and extends upward along the spine to the seventh chakra at the crown of your head and beyond. The masculine parts of the seven traditional chakras are connected to it.

**Gunas:** The masters of tantra used the gunas to describe the flavor of fields of energy fields with individual qualities. The Sanskrit word *guna* means "quality or attribute." In classical tantra there are three gunas: Sattva, Ragas, and Tamas.

**Hara:** Your strong center in your physical body. Hara is located four fingers width below your navel and about one inch (four centimeters) forward from your spine. In Japanese, the word *Hara* means abdomen. Taoists believe that Hara is the place in your physical body where you can find the elixir of life. It is also the place where you can reclaim your powerful center in your physical body.

**Healing space:** See woman's healing space.

**Inner beauty:** Has four essential aspects: good health, character, inner peace, and prana.

**Inner peace:** Inner peace is a state of stillness that emerges from deep within you. It emerges when movement stops and you can focus your mind on the joy that spontaneously radiates through your energy field.

**Intent:** A function of your authentic mind that is active on all worlds and dimensions of the physical and non-physical universe. You can use your intent to program your mental attention to locate a concentration of karmic baggage or an attachment that is responsible for a physical ailment or self-limiting pattern.

**Interdimensional being:** Any sentient being that has both physical and non-physical vehicles. Humans are interdimensional beings.

**Intrusions:** Created by the violent projection of distorted energy with individual qualities into a person's subtle energy field. They produce self-limiting and anti-self patterns.

**Karma:** Sanskrit word that comes from the root *kri*, "to act," and it signifies an activity or action. In the West, karma has been defined as the cumulative effect of action, which is commonly expressed as "You reap what you sow."

**Karmic baggage:** Dense energy with individual qualities. In your energy field, karmic baggage creates pressure and muscle ache when you're stressed, and it creates self-limiting and anti-self patterns that produce anxiety, self-doubt, and confusion. It's the main obstacle to the experience of radiant good health and transcendent relationship.

**Karmic pattern:** Energetic patterns created by attachments and by the accumulation of karmic baggage in the subtle energy field. These patterns create behavior that is self-limiting and disruptive to power, creativity, and radiance.

**Karmic wounds:** An energetic wound caused by an energetic trauma; see karmic baggage.

**Kundalini-Shakti:** Greatest repository of prana in your energy field; emerged from Shakti, via the tattvas, along with you and everything else in the phenomenal universe; comes in two forms: structural Kundalini and the serpent energy, which is located at the base of the spine.

**Life-affirming archetypes:** These are archetypes that support a person's power, creativity, and radiance. They promote dharma and they make life more joyful by promoting the flow of prana.

**Life-affirming identity:** One that has as its foundation self-confidence, self-esteem, and empathy for others.

**Life-affirming qualities:** The foundation of a person's power, creativity, and radiance. These qualities include pleasure, love, intimacy, and joy as well as the qualities of good character. See character.

**Light body field:** A resource field with a vibration one step higher than the core field. Like the core field, it fills your energy field and physical body—and extends beyond it in all directions. By enhancing the functions of the light body field and centering yourself in it, you will find a place within your soul where lust is superseded by authentic passion and your authentic feminine qualities emerge without distortion.

**Manas:** See aspects of mind.

**Matriarchal society:** In matriarchal societies, lineage passes through the mother. Because lineage passes through the mother, the core values of matriarchy enhance the balance of male-female forces in women and men as well as in the institutions of society. This leads to a balanced, non-violent society that values life and relationships above power and wealth.

**Meridians:** Part of your energy system; streams of energy that transfer prana from the chakras to the energetic vehicles and auric fields. The flow of energy with universal qualities through the meridians enables a person to remain centered in their authentic mind, to form an authentic identity, and to participate in transcendent relationship.

**Middle way:** A balanced life that includes empathy and the power to express yourself and the universal qualities of the feminine freely. By embracing the middle way, a woman will be able to perform as well as a man—or even better—in any job or productive activity because she will have enough power and energy to support her progress and guarantee her success.

**Mind:** The mind is composed of three essential elements. On the physical level, it includes the brain and nervous system as well as the chemicals in the body, including hormones that influence its structure and activities.

On the non-physical level, the mind includes the subtle energy field, its organs, and vehicles—and the prana that nourishes them. The combination of physical and non-physical elements creates the third part of the human mind—the network. The network includes the connections the mind has to its individual parts and to things beyond itself. This includes consciousness and energy—as well as attachments to other people, non-physical beings and their projections.

**Minor energy centers:** Part of your energy system; located throughout your body. Four principle centers are located in the extremities—one in each hand and one in each foot. Others are scattered throughout your energy field. Their principle function is to facilitate the movement of prana through your subtle energy field and physical body.

**Mudra:** Symbolic gesture which can be made with the hands and fingers or in combination with the tongue and feet. Each mudra has a specific affect on the human energy field and the energy flowing through it.

**Mutual field of prana:** Partners can create a field of energy with universal qualities that fills them and surrounds them both. That field, which we call the mutual field of prana, will be strong enough to prevent karmic baggage and restrictive beliefs from interfering with their experience of intimacy.

**Negative ions:** Created in nature as air molecules break apart due to sunlight, moving air, and water. They're odorless, tasteless, and invisible molecules that we inhale in abundance in certain environments. Think mountains, waterfalls, and beaches. Once they reach our bloodstream, negative ions are believed to produce biochemical reactions that increase the levels of the mood-enhancing chemical serotonin. It's believed that enhanced serotonin levels help alleviate depression, relieve stress, and boost energy—all of which enhance health and beauty.

**Neglect:** A woman can experience the trauma of neglect if her parents or guardians don't want her, if they want a boy, or if they're too self-involved to care for her properly. Neglect always involves the rejection of the child psychologically and energetically.

**Ohm:** The cosmic sound. It emerged when the universe was created. Its therapeutic effect is well known especially when it's used with the appropriate meditations and mudras.

**Orgasmic bliss:** An enduring condition, deep within your energy field, created through the union of consciousness (Shiva) and energy with universal qualities (Shakti). The merging of consciousness and energy provides you with a safe haven, deep within you, where you already experience oneness and where nothing can interfere with your experience of transcendent relationship.

**Passive aggressive patterns:** Energetic patterns used by people who feel powerless and cannot assert their power freely. They're self-limiting and are commonly found in rigid societies that don't honor the universal qualities of the feminine. Passive aggressive patterns manifest themselves in relationship games such as nagging, seduction, and guilt trips.

**Past life lover:** A lover from a past life to whom you are still attached. Attachments to past life lovers can create a yearning for one or more of their qualities and this can disrupt your subtle energy field and your intimate relationships.

**Personal healing space:** See woman's healing space.

**Polarity:** The degree to which your energy field is polarized masculine or feminine. The principle of polarity, as defined by *The Kybalion*, is that "Everything is dual; everything has poles; everything has its pair of opposites; like and unlike are the same; opposites are identical in nature, but different in degree; extremes meet; all truths are but half truths; all paradoxes may be reconciled."

**Prakriti field:** The field of prakriti is a resource field that contains some of the highest and purest frequencies of feminine energy. Like all resource fields, the prakriti field fills your energy field and extends beyond it in all directions.

**Prana bandage:** Will have a profound impact on your psychological health and the health of your energy field because it will seal the energetic wound created by a miscarriage, stillbirth, or abortion.

**Purusha field:** The primordial masculine field. It's a resource field that emerged along with the field of prakriti, the primordial field of feminine energy, during the fourth tattva, the fourth step in the evolution of the universe.

**Ragistic energy:** Less dense than tamasic energy. In most cases, ragistic energy will have less impact on your health and well-being. But the presence of an inordinate amount of ragistic energy will push you out of your strong center and make it difficult for you to embrace the universal qualities of the feminine; see gunas.

**Raja yoga:** The yoga of power and energy. One of the four classical yogas.

**Resonance:** The vibration or mean frequency that is the signature of a field of energy or living being. Every living being and/or field of energy with individual or universal qualities has its own resonance.

**Resource field:** A field of consciousness and/or energy with universal qualities that nourishes your energy field and the energetic vehicles within it. Resource fields are almost infinite in size and both fill and surround your energy field.

**Restrictive belief:** Any belief accepted as true by an institution of society, which prevents people from expressing themselves freely. Restrictive beliefs restrict the flow of prana and make it difficult for people to stay centered in their energy fields.

**Restrictive belief systems:** Restrict the flow of prana through your subtle energy system; they validate self-limiting patterns and in extreme cases can even contribute to the creation of obsessions, which can cause anti-self and anti-social behavior.

**Sattvic energy:** Less dense than either tamasic or ragistic energy. This makes it less disruptive to human health and well-being. However, it can still separate you from your strong center in your physical body and subtle energy field. And it can make it difficult for you to be yourself and express yourself freely. See gunas.

**Scold's bridle:** The scold's bridle was a metal and leather device that fit over the mouth and was fixed in the back. It had a tongue depressor with spurs or sharp edges. When it went into the woman's mouth, it made talking painful. The device was meant to humiliate a woman convicted by a council of men for nagging.

**Self-limiting archetypes:** A distorted and/or superficial image of a person that limits their power, creativity, and radiance. It does this by distorting their feelings about their body and their personality—and by making it difficult for a person to create a healthy life-affirming identity.

**Sheaths:** Interpenetrate your physical body like energy bodies; composed of energy with universal qualities; allow you to interact directly with your external environment and other sentient beings; give you the flexibility to express yourself and to participate in transcendent relationship.

**Shiva/Shakti:** Shiva and Shakti are revered as both the divine couple and as the archetypes for consciousness (Shiva) and energy (Shakti).

**Silver cord:** Each energy body is connected to the energy field of a person by a silver cord that extends from the back of the neck and can stretch almost indefinitely.

**Standard Method:** Takes about twenty minutes. In the first part, you relax the major muscle groups of your physical body by contracting and releasing them. In the second part, you use your intent to turn your organs of perception inward so that you can locate and stay centered in your subtle energy field.

**Subtle energy field:** Your energy field contains energetic vehicles that allow you to express yourself and interact with your environment on both the physical and non-physical levels. It also contains resource fields and a subtle energy system that supplies your energy field with life-affirming, feminine energy.

**Subtle energy system:** Your subtle energy system includes the chakra gates and chakra fields, meridians, auras, and minor energy centers scattered through your subtle energy field. In the same way that an electrical grid provides energy to homes and businesses, the organs of your subtle energy system transmit and transmute all the prana your physical body and your energetic vehicles need to function healthfully.

**Surface boundaries:** Your surface boundaries are the surfaces of your energy fields. They surround all of your energy fields (auras and resource fields) and your energetic vehicles. A person with weak surface boundaries will feel insecure and won't be able to fully manifest the universal qualities of the feminine.

**Tamasic energy:** The most dense and distorted form of energy with individual qualities. When there is an inordinate amount of tamasic energy trapped in your subtle energy field, it will cause the most distress and will have the most disruptive effect on your health and well-being. See gunas.

**Tantra/tantrics:** An ancient school of Indian thought which views energy with universal qualities and consciousness as essentially the same. Shiva who represents consciousness and Shakti who represents energy were depicted in tantric iconography in eternal embrace, which means that they are considered fundamentally the same.

**Tattvas:** Steps in the evolutionary process. The word combines the Sanskrit root *tat* which means "that," and *tvam*, which means "thou" or "you." Thus tattva signifies the ancient truth that you are always in union with Universal Consciousness and that you can experience the benefits of union (which include pleasure, love, intimacy, and joy) by remaining centered in your authentic mind. According to yoga and tantra, evolution in the physical and non-physical universe has gone through thirty-six steps already.

**Third heart:** See three hearts.

**Third heart field:** A resource field. It's through the third heart field that you will experience transcendent relationship with yourself and with the people you love.

**Three hearts:** Each person has three hearts—the physical heart on the left side of their chest, the heart chakra in the center of their chest, and *Atman*—the third heart on the right site of their chest. It's from Atman that bliss emerges into your conscious awareness.

**Traditional relationship:** In traditional relationships, women are expected to support their husbands, sacrifice their own needs for the sake of their loved ones, and transmit the core values of their society to their children.

**Transcendence:** The state of union or intimacy with Universal Consciousness, yourself and your partner. In the transcendent state, you can experience and share bliss and the universal qualities of pleasure, love, intimacy, and joy without disruption.

**Transcendent relationship:** A relationship where partners can share pleasure, love, intimacy, and joy without blockages, karmic baggage, or anything else getting in the way. Traditional relationship is about living within limitations. In contrast, a transcendent relationship is about transcending limitations, which is why in a transcendent relationship a radiant woman will experience a satisfaction unavailable to women in traditional relationships.

**Trauma:** Every traumatic event includes two traumas, a physical-psychological trauma and a subtle energetic trauma that is non-physical—but no less real. It's the violence done to the subtle energy field that is responsible for the most acute and enduring symptoms the survivor must endure.

**Universal consciousness:** Singularity that combines all aspects of the feminine and masculine; yin-yang. It's the foundation of your authentic mind as well as everything else in the physical and non-physical universe, including time, space, energy, and consciousness.

**Universal feminine:** Motivates humans to unite and to experience intimacy with one another. It makes everybody a healer, a lover—and on the deepest level a radiant, transcendent being—who has the capacity to transform the world through their work and relationships.

**Universal qualities:** Universal qualities include pleasure, love, intimacy, and joy as well as truth and freedom. Universal qualities do not create attachments—they support dharma, transcendent relationship, and self-realization.

**Vehicle:** An energetic vehicle. You have two types of energetic vehicles, energy bodies and sheaths. Energy bodies allow you to be present and sheaths allow you to interact with other sentient beings.

**Woman's healing space:** Something a woman creates within her energy field. It's a place where she can use her healing skills to heal her body, soul, and spirit and to do the same for the people she loves. To create your healing space, you must combine the energy and consciousness of two resource fields, the field of Prakriti and the field of Empathy.

**Yang Yu meridians:** The two Yang Yu meridians are your masculine arm channels located in both arms. They link your shoulders with the energy centers in your palms, after passing through the middle fingers.

**Yin/Yang:** Yin represents femininity, body, soul, earth, moon, water, night, cold, darkness, and contraction. Yang is masculine, mental, spirit, heaven, sun, day, fire, heat, sunlight, and expansion.

**Yin Yu meridians:** Feminine arm channels that link the centers in the palms with the chest. They travel along the insides of each arm. Along with the two Yang Yu meridians, they form the minor energy centers in the palms.

**Yoga:** Union. It also refers to an ancient scientific method developed in India to achieve enlightenment.

**Yogic breath:** A yogic breathing technique; by breathing yogically you will restore your breathing to its natural state and enhance the level of prana that radiates through your energy field.

**Yoni:** Sanskrit word that means "divine passage" or "place of birth."
On the physical level, it corresponds to a woman's vagina. In a wider
context, it also means origin, fountain, or sacred space: the space occupied by a radiant woman in her fullness, both as the manifestation
of the universal feminine and as the wellspring of sexual pleasure.

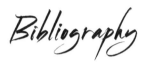

# Bibliography

Boakye, Priscilla Akua. "DIPO-Puberty Rites Among the Krobos of Eastern Region, Ghana." University of Tromsø, Project 2009/1415-2, Master Programme in Indigenous Studies.

Cummings, E. E. "A Poet's Advice to Students" in *A Miscellany*. Edited by George J. Firmage. New York: Argophile Press, 1958.

DiMaria, Lauren. "Children are More Prone to Depression During Puberty." About.com. Updated August 27, 2011. http://depression. about.com/od/teenchild/a/depression-during-puberty.htm.

Fisher, Helen F. *The Sex Contract: The Evolution of Human Behavior*. New York: William Morrow, 1983.

Goethe, Johann Wolfgang von. "Die Braut von Korinth." Tuebingen, Germany: Cotta Verlag, 1798.

Hänsel, Rudolf. "Die zu häufige Nutzung digitaler Medien vermindert die geistige Leistungsfähigkeit unserer Kinder." October 2012. http://www.zeit-fragen.ch/index.php?id=1170.

Howe Gaines, Janet. "Lilith in the Bible, Art and Mythology." Biblical Archaeology Society. Updated August 11, 2014. http://www.biblicalarchaeology.org/daily/people-cultures-in-the-bible/people-in-the-bible/lilith/.

Humm, Alan. "Overview of Lilith." http://jewishchristianlit.com/
Topics/Lilith/.

Jones, Adam. "Case Study: The European Witch-Hunts, c. 1450-1750."
Gendercide.org. http://www.gendercide.org/case_witchhunts.
html.

Lysebeth, Andre van. *Tantra*. Munich: Mosaik Verlag, 1990.

McCarthy, Wendy Ann. *Ich bin Bewusstsein*. Zwickau D: Innenwelt
Verlag, 2013.

Miyoshi, Shunichiro. "Menstrual Blood Shows Heart Repairing Stem
Cell Properties." Medical News Today. Updated April 25, 2008.
http://www.medicalnewstoday.com/articles/105322.php.

Mumford, John. *Ecstasy Through Tantra*. St. Paul, MN: Llewellyn Publications, 1975.

Pro Femina e.V. "Komplikationen nach einer oder mehrerer Abtreibun-
gen." http://www.vorabtreibung.net/node/43.

Pröll, Gabriele. *Das Geheimnis der Menstruation, Kraft und Weisheit des
Mondzyklus*. Munich: Goldmann Verlag, 2004.

St. Hieronymus. "Women are unclean during Menstruation." http://
www.womenpriests.org/de/traditio/unclean.asp#latin.

Stiene, Bronwen, and Frans Stiene. "The Deeper Meaning of Hara."
Shibumi International Reiki Association (blog). http://www.shibu-
mireiki.org.

Swamini Mayatitananda. "Honoring Shakti." www.organickarma.
co.uk/shakti-energy.html.

Tjaden, Patricia, and Nancy Thoennes. "Full Report of the Prevalence,
Incidence, and Consequences of Violence Against Women." Cre-
ateSpace Independent Publishing Platform, 1998.

Trieb, Traude. Kindlein Komm Tee. www.traude-trieb.at.

Walker, Barbara G. *Das Geheime Wissen der Frauen*. German edition of
*The Woman's Encyclopedia of Myths and Secrets*. Uhlstädt-Kirchhasel:
Arun-Verlag, 2007.

Wolf, Doris. "Sex ohne sexuelle Phantasien geht nicht." http://www.
partnerschaft-beziehung.de/sex-gehirn.html.

# Recommended Reading

Jnana Yoga, by Swami Vividananda

Tripura Rahasya—The Mystery Behind the Trinity

The Dhammapada

The Kybalion

The Bhagavad Gita

Tao Te Ching

A Woman's Encyclopedia of Myths and Secrets, by Barbara G. Walker

Kundalini Yoga, by Swami Sivanananda

# Index